Raising a Child
With Arthritis

A PARENT'S GUIDE

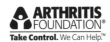

ARTHRITIS
FOUNDATION®
Take Control. We Can Help.™

THIS BOOK HAS BEEN REVIEWED BY INDEPENDENT MEDICAL
EXPERTS. THE ARTHRITIS FOUNDATION THANKS AMGEN AND WYETH
FOR UNDERWRITING THE DEVELOPMENT OF THIS BOOK.

AMGEN® Wyeth®

Raising a Child
With Arthritis

A PARENT'S GUIDE

. . . .

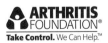

AN OFFICIAL PUBLICATION OF THE ARTHRITIS FOUNDATION

ATLANTA, GEORGIA

Printed in the Canada

This book is not intended as a substitute for the medical advice of physicians.

Published by:
Arthritis Foundation
1330 West Peachtree Street, Suite 100
Atlanta, GA 30309

Library of Congress Card Catalog Number: 2008928989

ISBN: 978-0-912423-55-5

The mission of the Arthritis Foundation is to improve lives through leadership in the
prevention, control and cure of arthritis and related diseases.

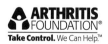

The information in this book does not cover all possible uses, actions, precautions, side
effects or interactions of the treatments used to treat juvenile arthritis. It should not replace
the advice and guidance given by your child's doctor. If you have questions regarding your
child's disease or treatment, ask your doctor or pharmacist. The Arthritis Foundation does not
endorse any brand-name or generic medication.

Table of Contents

Table of Contents

Acknowledgments

This book wouldn't have been possible without the time and assistance of the following people, who provided their clinical expertise, suggested materials and assisted in many ways: Beth Axtell, research communications specialist, Arthritis Foundation; Wade Balmer, director, operations and mission integration, Arthritis Foundation Eastern Pennsylvania Chapter; Elizabeth Compton, vice president, publishing, Arthritis Foundation; Edward H. Giannini, MSc, DrPH, professor of pediatrics, University of Cincinnati College of Medicine; Michael Henrickson, MD, clinical associate professor and clinical director, pediatric rheumatology at the University of Oklahoma College of Medicine; Christie Jarrett, publishing assistant, Arthritis Foundation; James Jarvis, MD, professor of pediatrics and section chief, pediatric rheumatology at the University of Oklahoma College of Medicine; Susan Klepper, PhD, PT, assistant professor of clinical physical therapy, Columbia University; Carol B. Lindsley, MD, professor of pediatrics and chief of pediatric rheumatology at University of Kansas Medical Center; Daniel J. Lovell, MD, MPH, Joseph E. Levinson professor of pediatric rheumatology, Cincinnati Children's Hospital Medical Center; Amy Melnick, MPA, chief public policy officer, Arthritis Foundation; Sampath Prahalad MD, MSc, assistant professor of pediatrics, University of Utah School of Medicine; Marilynn G. Punaro, MD, director, Arthritis Services, Texas Scottish Rite Hospital; Michael A. Rapoff, PhD, professor and chief of behavioral pediatrics at University of Kansas Medical Center; Laura Robbins, DSW, vice president of education and academic affairs at the Hospital for Special Surgery, New York City; Eric Schiffman, DDS, MS, director of the TMD and Orofacial Pain Division at the University of Minnesota's School of Dentistry; Danielle Stephens, director, Community Development and Camp JRA, Arthritis Foundation Eastern Pennsylvania Chapter; Carol A. Wallace, MD, professor of pediatrics, Division of Rheumatology, University of Washington and Children's Hospital and Medical Center; and Patience H. White, MD, MA, chief public health officer, Arthritis Foundation.

. . . .

A special thank you goes to Harry L. Gewanter, MD, FAAP, FACR, pediatric rheumatologist, Richmond, Virginia; Dawn Hafeli, vice president for programs, Arthritis Foundation Michigan Chapter; and Susan Wright, OT, research assistant and occupational therapist at Kansas University Medical Center in the Department of Pediatrics, who shared their time so generously.

. . . .

This book was written by Charlotte Huff and medically edited by Richard Vehe, MD. The editorial directors of this book were Bethany Afshar and Robin Yamakawa. The book was designed by Donald Partyka. The book cover was designed by Ibiyomi Jegede. The creative director of this book was Audrey Wiederstein.

About the Author and Editor

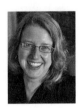

Charlotte Huff has written about health and parenting issues for more than 15 years, working for daily newspapers and writing for national magazines. Her feature writing includes articles for *American Baby, Arthritis Today, Current Health* and *Southwest Spirit*, among others. She lives in Fort Worth, Texas, with her husband and young son.

. . . .

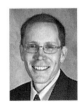

Richard K. Vehe, MD, is director of the Division of Pediatric Rheumatology for the Department of Pediatrics at the University of Minnesota in Minneapolis, and the medical director for the Center for Pediatric Rheumatology at Gillette Children's Specialty Healthcare in St. Paul, Minn. He also is the medical editor of the Arthritis Foundation's newsletter for families of children with juvenile arthritis, *Kids Get Arthritis Too.*

Introduction

Until your child was diagnosed, you might never have realized that arthritis could strike the youngest among us. You likely had never administered an injection, or knew what a 504 plan was, or even knew what a pediatric rheumatologist did. And you probably had seldom before felt so angry, so helpless and so zealous to do anything to make your child feel better.

Whether your child was diagnosed last week, last year, or a decade ago, your family's path in life has been forever changed by arthritis. In this journey, you're following in the footsteps of thousands of parents before you. Nearly 300,000 children in the United States live with one of the many rheumatic diseases that fall under the umbrella of juvenile arthritis. The diagnosis is one of the most common in childhood, although it's still surprisingly, and frustratingly, unfamiliar to many people.

There's plenty of reason for optimism. Children who develop symptoms today benefit from more information and more tools than children diagnosed just a generation ago. Powerful medications have been developed, along with an increasingly sophisticated understanding of how they should be used to relieve your child's pain and inflammation. Ten years ago, when the Arthritis Foundation published the first edition of this book, the biologic treatment etanercept (*Enbrel*) had just been federally approved, the first in a new class of drugs for rheumatic diseases. Now doctors can select from a widening array of treatments, with additional drugs in the pipeline for possible approval in the next few years. By using those drugs earlier and more aggressively in the disease process, physicians strive to halt symptoms in their tracks, or at least to slow their progression to shield young joints from the permanent damage that was, in the past, a hallmark of this disease.

Long gone are the days when children with arthritis spent too many hours indoors, discouraged from exercising or playing with other kids, the disease limiting their movements and the expectation of what they could accomplish. Now therapists and physicians encourage children to remain as active as they can, without going overboard. With your support and advocacy, your child can pursue her passions on the athletic field, in the classroom, at summer camp, on family trips and beyond in life.

Raising a Child With Arthritis will not only answer some of your questions related to diagnosis and medications, but also will lay out what's understood about physical fitness, psychological aspects and school-related rights for kids with arthritis. You'll be provided numerous resources: exercises, checklists, Web site addresses and an appendix rich with other practical information.

You'll also read the stories of those living with the disease, along with their parents' perspectives on a variety of topics. You'll read about Wade Balmer's reflections on his own adolescent rebellion, Tracy Freeman's struggle to give her daughter a shot and Kerry Ludlam's experiences in dealing with gaps in health insurance. Through these pages, you'll witness children and young adults triumph in the classroom and athletics, swim competitively, advocate in the nation's capital, and reflect on their first year of motherhood. In all, you'll find their challenges are very familiar and that their accomplishments are inspiring. That they also happen to have been diagnosed with arthritis is often just a footnote.

. . . .

Note: We understand that both girls and boys get juvenile arthritis. However, for ease of use, we again used female pronouns throughout this edition.

Juvenile Arthritis: A Primer

Juvenile arthritis is essentially an umbrella term, designed to encompass the various diseases that typically involve some type of inflammatory component in children. In this section, we will discuss some of the more common types of juvenile arthritis and how the study of genetics is providing insights into these complex diseases. You will meet the many participants on your child's health-care team and learn more about the ongoing shortage of pediatric rheumatologists. And you'll get some grounding in treatment goals, particularly what's understood about achieving remission and preventing flares.

CHAPTER ONE

Getting Diagnosed: Steps and Obstacles

A nagging fatigue. A faint pinkish rash. A throbbing knee. A stubborn fever. A swollen hand.

Pain and swelling can flare unexpectedly one day, nearly immobilizing your once-active child as you shuttle between specialists, searching for answers. Or symptoms may be difficult to detect initially. Your child, particularly if she's quite young, may not recognize her discomfort as anything unusual. Or, she may adjust her activities and movements in ways that can be difficult to spot. She may rise more slowly from bed following a nap. You may one day realize that you can't recall the last time she jumped around the house, rattling the furniture. Something just doesn't seem ... normal.

You are not alone.

Nearly 300,000 American children are currently diagnosed with a form of juvenile arthritis or an arthritis-related condition, living with some degree of pain and discomfort. That's more children than those affected by Type 1 diabetes, and many more — at least four times more — than those diagnosed with sickle cell anemia or muscular dystrophy, diseases that are much more widely known and discussed in the media. Children also can develop arthritis related to other autoimmune diseases, such as lupus.

Children as young as 2, or even younger, may have juvenile arthritis.

Pediatric rheumatologists, the subspecialists that treat children with arthritis, work in a complex discipline which encompasses a multitude of inflammatory and noninflammatory disorders involving the connective tissues and joints. Common estimates hold that some 100 rheumatic diseases affect children. Depending upon the underlying diagnosis, symptoms can range from limited arthritis in a single joint to a system-wide inflammatory condition that can involve blood vessels and vital organs, along with the joints.

As a result, your journey from that first nagging worry — that parental instinct that something is wrong — to a firm diagnosis can feel serpentine indeed, slowed by a number of factors.

In some regions of the United States, pediatric rheumatologists are scarce, making it difficult to schedule a timely appointment. (*See sidebar, opposite page.*) Sometimes, your child's symptoms may have receded before a doctor's visit, only to re-emerge weeks or months later. Those symptoms can be the first clues to a number of other, similar illnesses, including those caused by infections (e.g., Lyme disease, acute rheumatic fever) and other causes.

Arthritis in children, to a large extent, is a diagnosis of omission. To identify the underlying illness, doctors must sift through and exclude other diagnoses first, a time-consuming process. Your child will likely have undergone a variety of laboratory and imaging tests, along with a detailed physical examination, before your doctor can provide any clear-cut answers.

Searching for Answers

No single blood test confirms juvenile arthritis. In fact, blood testing will reveal relatively little in terms of your child's diagnosis. (Although blood results may provide some insights into the future course of the disease, once your child is diagnosed.) Blood tests used in diagnosing adults with arthritis may not be as relevant in children. Few children, for example, test positive for a substance called rheumatoid factor, seen as a common marker for rheumatoid arthritis. This blood test is considered more helpful in diagnosing adult rheumatoid arthritis and classifying the severity of disease.

In children, the key to diagnosis is conducting a careful physical exam along with your child's medical history. By examining your child, sometimes

Where Are The Pediatric Rheumatologists?

If you've spent an entire day taking your child to the doctor, you're sharing the road with a lot of other parents.

Thirty-five percent of children live more than 50 miles from a pediatric rheumatologist, a physician with specialized training in treating children with rheumatic diseases, according to a landmark 2007 report by the U.S. Department of Health & Human Services, highlighting the serious shortage of these specialists. Nearly one in five children with arthritis must travel more than 100 miles to see such a specialist.

To meet the demand, at least 337 more pediatric rheumatologists are needed nationally — a 75 percent increase over the current number. Some states — as many as 13 in recent years — don't have any practicing pediatric rheumatologists within their boundaries.

What gives? Admittedly, pediatric rheumatology is a relatively new subspecialty. Board certification wasn't even offered until the early 1990s. Training programs are still catching up. Roughly one-third of medical schools and 40 percent of pediatric residency programs don't have pediatric rheumatologists available to educate physicians in training. For their part, pediatric rheumatologists point to the comparatively low salaries given the long working hours as a reason for the shortage. Since a substantial number of pediatric rheumatologists work in academic medical centers, they often handle teaching and other responsibilities, along with patient care.

Thankfully, steps are being taken to expand that vital pool of expertise. In recent years, the Arthritis Foundation has been advocating for the passage of the Arthritis Prevention, Control and Cure Act, which would, among other measures, encourage doctors to train in pediatric rheumatology by creating incentives, such as an education loan repayment program. Families are pitching in, too. In Alabama, a state without any pediatric rheumatologists for a stretch, a grassroots fundraising effort led by the local Arthritis Foundation office helped attract two pediatric rheumatologists to the state in 2007.

So what should you do if the closest pediatric rheumatologist practices several hours away? Well, like many parents, you simply insert the key into the ignition and start driving, or you seek alternatives. Start by networking with local families, through the Arthritis Foundation and other groups, to learn more about options closer to home. Perhaps a nearby pediatrician has accrued some clinical experience with juvenile arthritis or an adult rheumatologist also treats a significant number of children. Alternatively, you could use a two-pronged approach, visiting a long-distance specialist once or twice a year. Then for the checkups in between, you could consult a local doctor who can tap the expertise of the pediatric rheumatologist if anything unusual crops up.

in just the first few minutes, the physician will be able to identify the impact of inflammation on her joints.

First, let's learn a little detail about the joints themselves. A joint is the area where two bones meet. In healthy joints, a number of tissues help cushion and ease fluidity of motion. Cartilage covers the ends of the bones, and the joint is surrounded by a protective capsule that is lined with the synovium, a tissue that lubricates and nourishes the cartilage and bones within.

When inflammation strikes, that protective balance of cartilage, fluid and tissue is tipped. The synovium becomes inflamed. Your child may feel warmth and pain in the affected areas, and you may detect visible redness and swelling around the joint. The fluid, typically present in small quantities in normal joints, starts to overproduce.

Joint by Joint

During the physical exam, the doctor will feel your child's joints, one by one, searching for signs of fluid or swollen tissue. When affected, her joints might feel more squishy or spongy to the touch. Fluid building around a finger joint, when pressed, might feel much like squeezing a grape.

Sometimes fluid accumulation is easily visible; too much above the knee cap can make one thigh significantly larger than the other. Sometimes the signs can be more subtle. The area around your child's knee cap, instead of being concave, may look more filled in. By using a common scale to judge the level of swelling in joints, your doctor can rate the degree of your child's swelling, depending on how difficult it is to detect the bones in the affected joint.

The types of swelling also can vary, depending upon the arthritis involved. In an arthritis-related disease called systemic lupus erythematosus (SLE, or commonly called lupus), the swelling may be less obvious.

A JOINT ANATOMY PRIMER

Arthritis attacks the most important components of body mechanics – your joints, from cartilage to tendons. To better understand how treatment and medication works, it's important to understand the basic structure of how your child's joints connect and move:

Joint: The juncture where two bones meet.

Cartilage: The smooth gliding material that covers the bones.

Ligaments: Fibrous cords that attach one bone to the next, helping to stabilize the joints during movement.

Tendons: Much like ligaments, except they connect muscles to bone, acting like pulleys to move the joint.

Capsule: The tough material attached to the bones enclosing the joint cavity.

Synovium: The tissue lining the joint capsule, which can become thickened and can produce extra fluid when arthritis causes inflammation.

Synovial fluid: Produced by the synovium, it helps to nourish and lubricate the surface of the joint.

HEALTHY JOINT

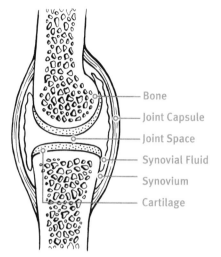

- Bone
- Joint Capsule
- Joint Space
- Synovial Fluid
- Synovium
- Cartilage

JOINT WITH RHEUMATOID ARTHRITIS

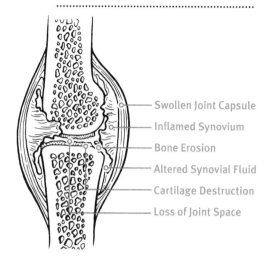

- Swollen Joint Capsule
- Inflamed Synovium
- Bone Erosion
- Altered Synovial Fluid
- Cartilage Destruction
- Loss of Joint Space

In another disease, psoriatic arthritis, it can involve both the tendons, which run along the length of the fingers or toes, as well as the joints themselves, until the child's digits swell to look like sausages.

Over time, your child may have modified her movements to minimize discomfort, rather than complain about it or even tell you about it. It's not that she doesn't feel the pain. Instead, she may not realize to what degree it has affected her personal body mechanics — similar to how a child may not realize the extent of her vision problems until sliding on that first pair of glasses. For that reason, your child's doctor will closely observe her movements and interactions in the examining room. If she is a toddler, how does she reach for a parent? How does she position her body when picked up? If your child is older, the doctor will scrutinize how she lifts herself onto the examining table. Does she avoid bending her wrists, instead balling her hands into fists and placing her weight there? These signs of modified behavior can tell the doctor a great deal about how she may be affected by pain.

The doctor also will check your child's range of movement for each joint, to make sure that arthritis isn't limiting the motion of joints or causing pain with motion. Sometimes, the doctor will pick up important

JOINT INFLAMMATION: SOME WARNING SIGNS

- Pain
- Swelling
- Warmth
- Limitation of movement
- Tenderness to the touch or pain with movement
- Stiffness after rest
- Pink or red skin

PERSONAL STORY

THE JOURNEY TO DIAGNOSIS
Corey Mayfield's Story

Corey Mayfield's family first began to worry when the 6-year-old girl complained of ankle pain after her Irish dance class. A small, red lump had appeared on her left ankle, one that was surprisingly warm to the touch, Corey's mother, Jenn, recalls. "I just assumed that it was a bruise and it had swelled a little bit," she says.

They consulted one doctor and then another, followed by yet another. Before Corey was diagnosed with juvenile arthritis, she saw several specialists and was fitted for two casts. The first doctor thought the problem was a ganglion cyst and set a cast. The second doctor yelled at Mayfield for over-scheduling her daughter—Corey also was playing soccer and lacrosse at the time—and diagnosed tendinitis. Corey was fitted for a second cast and ordered to rest the joint.

It was the third doctor, an orthopedic surgeon, who first raised the possibility of juvenile arthritis, along with Lyme disease. He gave Corey a cortisone shot and advised a wait-and-see stance. Soon after, Corey complained bitterly of knee pain while sitting in a movie theater. Mayfield leaned over in the dark and rested a hand on her daughter's knee.

It was warm to the touch and squishy feeling, almost like a wet sponge. "It seemed like we would never get the right diagnosis—that no one knew what they were talking about," she says. "It did seem like an eternity."

Now Mayfield realizes that the time they spent in diagnostic limbo—just two months from Corey's initial pain to a firm explanation—was practically warp speed, compared with what some families face.

In the years since, Corey has become a vocal advocate on the behalf of children living with chronic diseases, testifying before the Maryland House and Senate in favor of the passage of the Maryland Stem Cell Research Act. She still plays soccer, wrapping her knees in bandages if they are bothersome that day. By age 9, she was giving herself weekly methotrexate shots.

Before she gives each shot, her hand shakes. "She has to physically and emotionally work herself up," her mother says. But she insists on doing it herself. "She wants control over her destiny, her future—her health. She says, 'I've got to have control.'"

> **"It seemed like we would never get the right diagnosis."**

clues from just having fun with her — shaking her hand, wiggling her arms or clapping her feet together. To get a better sense of spontaneous motion, the doctor might tickle her, checking if her movements are fluid, rather than stiff or herky-jerky.

Another warning sign can be spotting something unusual in how your child walks, technically referred to as a gait disturbance. Depending on which joints are involved, your child may attempt to compensate by changing her walk. For example, if she can't fully extend her left knee, she might instead walk on the toes of her left foot. If her left hip is sore and stuck, she might swing the pelvis and leg forward together to take a step. Pain in the toes, where they meet the ball of the foot, also can affect walking. Rather than rolling forward on her foot to push off, your child may rely more on her heels.

BREAKING DOWN THE BLOOD WORK

In the course of diagnosis, your child will typically be scheduled for several blood tests. None will definitively diagnose arthritis, but they can rule out other potential causes of your child's symptoms, such as infections. Once your child is diagnosed, the results might provide some indication of the types of symptoms, or severity of disease, she could face in the years ahead. They may also be used to help tailor her treatments and monitor for side effects.

ANA (antinuclear antibody) test: This test looks for a protein, or antibody, made by white blood cells, that binds to the contents of a cell's nucleus, or central core. In children with some types of juvenile arthritis, this test can provide an indication of the long-term risk of developing a serious eye inflammation called uveitis.

CBC, or complete blood count: This test checks the red blood cells, white blood cells and platelets. Anemia, or a low red blood cell count, can occur with iron deficiency or with chronic inflammation, and can contribute to fatigue.

Chemistries: Your child may have other tests to check liver function, kidney function and other potential organ problems that could be causes of their symptoms.

ESR (erythrocyte sedimention rate), or "sed rate": This test provides an indication of inflammation in the body, although it is by no means conclusive. Someone with a normal sed rate can still have arthritis. Conversely, someone with a high sed rate may not appear to be seriously ill.

HLA (human leukocyte antigen)-B27: This test looks for a gene that's associated with arthritis that involves the spine, such as ankylosing spondylitis. Most children with this gene are healthy, but they are more likely than others to develop this arthritis. Your child can test negative and still have this form of arthritis diagnosed.

Rheumatoid factor test (RF): Frequently associated with rheumatoid arthritis in adults, this test also looks for an antibody made by the white blood cells. It's rarely positive in children unless they have developed a type of arthritis — RF-positive polyarthritis — that's equivalent to adult rheumatoid arthritis. Children and adults who test positive face a greater risk of severe disease and are often treated more aggressively with medications.

PERSONAL ESSAY
. . . .

HOW COULD I HAVE MISSED THAT?
Ann Huffman's Essay

Gazing at photographs of my daughter, Leslie, I see her story of juvenile arthritis played out in silent pictures. During those years, a sweetly rounded preschooler at age 3 became a painfully thin kindergartener by age 5. Six more years would go by before she was diagnosed with polyarticular arthritis.

Every time I look at a snapshot and see Leslie's swollen knuckles and wrists, I think, "How could I have missed that?"

I have a permanent video in my memory of Leslie walking like a stiff-legged little soldier when she'd get out of bed in the morning. She only gained two pounds in two years and had very little appetite.

"How could I have missed that?" Eventually we realized her wrists no longer bent backwards. "That's odd," I thought. For all those years, arthritis was flying under the radar.

Actually, I didn't miss any of those symptoms. I simply didn't know what they meant. When I questioned the pediatrician about the size of Leslie's joints the doctor reassured me they would look normal once Leslie gained a little weight. Since Leslie's older sister and brother were also slight in stature it seemed "normal" for Leslie to be tiny. My mother's instinct didn't agree. It was not until Leslie complained of jaw pain at age 11 that the red flag went up in the doctor's mind.

Fortunately we live in the Cleveland area with a pediatric rheumatologist only thirty minutes away. It took Leslie's doctor all of five minutes to diagnose what had taken years of disease to produce. And I asked him, "How could I have missed this?" In his no-nonsense way, he assured me I would have known if the arthritis had been in different joints such as hips and knees — she would have been limping. "Don't bother feeling guilty," he said. "It's an unproductive emotion."

Leslie is now working full-time and engaged to be married. Arthritis still plays a role in her life, but she doesn't let it get in the way of living. It may be on the radar screen now, but it's only a small blip in her very big life.

> "I didn't miss any of those symptoms. I simply didn't know what they meant."

—*Ann Huffman lives in Rocky River, Ohio. Her daughter Leslie is 25.*

CHAPTER ONE GETTING DIAGNOSED: STEPS AND OBSTACLES

Along with the physical exam itself, your child's doctors will take a number of other diagnostic steps, in part to rule out other potential causes of her symptoms. Blood work, for example, can rule out the possibility of an underlying infection. Among the diagnostic steps:

- **Medical history:** By asking questions, details can be gathered about the nature and duration of your child's symptoms. The doctor will also collect information about your child's family history to determine if any relatives have been diagnosed with arthritis or other autoimmune conditions, conditions where the child's immune system is affected or malfunctions for some reason. The doctor will ask other questions to gather clues to help identify possible causes for your child's symptoms.

- **Laboratory work:** Your doctor may order a battery of blood tests, which can help identify the cause of your child's symptoms, and importantly, exclude other illnesses that could mimic juvenile arthritis. For some types of arthritis, along with tests that search for antibodies, such as rheumatoid factor or antinuclear antibody, a complete blood count and urinalysis, or urine test, might be done.

- **X-rays and other imaging tests:** These tests are done to look for fractures, tumors, bone infections or other problems that can cause joint pain. Often, early X-rays of arthritis aren't informative, but over time, the X-ray pictures might reveal whether the arthritis is well controlled or is causing damage to the bone or joint cartilage. Other imaging tests may include bone scan, ultrasound, CT (computerized tomography) scan or MRI (magnetic resonance imaging).

More Than Pain Alone

You might associate pain with arthritis and assume it's one of the first reported symptoms. You're not alone. Pediatric rheumatologists frequently admit that too many doctors refer children to them based on complaints of pain and little else.

But pain is rarely a strong indicator that your child has juvenile arthritis, or really any rheumatic disease. In one study of 414 children, one-fourth of the children reported pain as their sole complaint, but only one of those children had any form of rheumatic disease. Of the 76 children eventually diagnosed with some type of juvenile arthritis, only 12 of them (16 percent) listed pain among their symptoms.

ARTHRITIS FOUNDATION **11**

The same study also validated the belief that blood tests contribute little in the diagnosis of juvenile arthritis. Neither the blood tests for rheumatoid factor or another antibody, antinuclear antibody (ANA), appear useful in this area. What diagnostic measures were helpful? Of those children ultimately diagnosed with juvenile rheumatoid arthritis, 72 percent complained of swelling in the joints, and nearly one in three had visible gait disturbances.

The Diagnostic Bottom Line

As you can see, diagnosis can be far from easy. Sometimes your child's doctor will be able to make a general diagnosis of juvenile arthritis, but will have to wait months to see how the symptoms unfold to more precisely identify the type, or to predict any type of long-term prognosis. In the systemic form of arthritis, for example, the first sign might be a worrisome fever, appearing before any joint inflammation.

In the years ahead, researchers hope that genetic breakthroughs will help them more quickly identify the underlying disease that is causing these troubling symptoms in children. For parents still awaiting a diagnosis, it's important to trust your parental instinct if you're not satisfied with the answers you're receiving regarding the cause of your child's pain or swelling. A second opinion is always an option, even if a lengthy drive is required to the nearest pediatric rheumatologist. The sooner a child is correctly diagnosed, the faster medication, exercise and other interventions can be started to combat inflammation and its long-term effects. ●

. . . .

CHAPTER TWO

Getting Specific: What Type?

Arthritis in children is nothing new. Physicians have been documenting cases of pain and inflammation in children for more than a century. Along with juvenile rheumatoid arthritis, medical textbooks also described symptoms that point to other types of rheumatic disease, including lupus and scleroderma.

Still, chronic arthritis in children didn't receive significant medical attention until the years following the discovery of the so-called "wonder drug," penicillin. As the antibiotic's usage became widespread in the mid-1900s, doctors were able nearly to wipe out acute rheumatic fever, a formerly terrifying condition. The medical community shifted its focus to children who suffered from forms of chronic inflammation. American hospitals, initially built to treat children with rheumatic fever, changed their focus as well. By the 1970s, pediatric rheumatology emerged more as a unique subspecialty, especially with the establishment of a pediatric arm of the American College of Rheumatology, the professional association of rheumatologists, and the first pediatric rheumatology conference in the United States.

And the field of pediatric rheumatology, along with its understanding of rheumatic diseases in children, continues to evolve. The dedicated professionals who treat these incredibly complex diseases in such young and vulnerable patients continue to revise the terms used to describe specific types of the disease and strive to find the right approach to treatment.

Juvenile arthritis, in short, is no more than a catchall term. There are many different autoimmune and inflammatory conditions that can develop before age 16. The word "arthritis" literally means joint inflammation: arth (joint) and itis (inflammation). In recent years, though, researchers have developed a more sophisticated understanding of the differences between the types of arthritis, and we now have more specific names for these challenging conditions.

New diagnoses have been identified through recent research. For example, Kawasaki disease, which involves inflammation of the walls of the blood vessels, was first described by a Japanese pediatrician in the 1960s.

Parents often want to know the exact diagnosis of their child's condition, and understanding the differences between these diseases may help parents sift through complicated medical news and information more effectively. Juvenile rheumatoid arthritis, or JRA, is the most common form of juvenile arthritis. The term JRA dates back more than 50 years in North America. Within the broad category of JRA, researchers specify a child's diagnosis primarily based on the number of joints involved. Children with arthritis in relatively few joints, four or less, were described as having pauciarticular arthritis. Children with a larger number of affected joints were diagnosed with the polyarticular form of the disease. Lately, you may have noticed another term — juvenile idiopathic arthritis — if you've been reading newer studies or have changed physicians recently.

More and more physicians are dropping the term "JRA" for a number of reasons. For one thing, juvenile

....

JUVENILE ARTHRITIS: GETTING A PRECISE COUNT

How many children have juvenile arthritis? It's hard to say exactly how many kids live with these diseases, mainly because experts disagree about which diagnoses should be included.

In one of the most comprehensive efforts to date, researchers at the Centers for Disease Control and Prevention analyzed diagnostic data to determine the number of children being treated for an arthritis-related condition during a four-year period. Besides identifying children with juvenile rheumatoid arthritis, they also captured data on other rheumatic diagnoses, including diseases of the connective tissues, scleroderma and ankylosing spondylitis, to name a few.

The results: An estimated 294,000 children annually were treated during the four years, from 2001 to 2004.

The impact on the health care system was substantial, the researchers reported in the December 2007 issue of *Arthritis Care & Research*. On average, those children visited a doctor a total of 827,000 times annually; their annual visits to the emergency department totaled 83,000.

rheumatoid arthritis is not — as the term implies — a pint-sized replica of rheumatoid arthritis in adults. It's believed that only about 10 percent of children have a disease that closely mirrors the adult disease. Also, as time has progressed, many researchers have concluded that the types of arthritis included under the JRA category were drawn too narrowly and should include some related diagnoses, such as ankylosing spondylitis.

As experts gained a better understanding of this group of diseases, they developed a new moniker: juvenile idiopathic arthritis. ("Idiopathic" means "of unknown origin." To this day, the exact cause of juvenile arthritis is still, unfortunately, unknown.) The term, first proposed by the International League of Associations for Rheumatology in the mid-1990s, is not exactly interchangeable with juvenile rheumatoid arthritis because it includes diagnoses that weren't part of the previous JRA definition.

As the term is more broadly adopted in the United States, you might encounter a sometimes confusing hodgepodge of terms and names. Older scientific studies, including some cited in this book, will classify disease based on the traditional JRA classifications — pauciarticular, polyarticular and systemic. Be sure to clarify which disease your child has with your physician if you're uncertain or confused about any of the terms being used.

The following sections outline how the types of juvenile idiopathic arthritis, as well as other arthritis-related conditions, are defined currently.

Juvenile Idiopathic Arthritis (JIA)

Considered the most common form of arthritis, juvenile idiopathic arthritis (JIA) begins before age 16. To be diagnosed, initial swelling in one or more joints must persist at least six weeks. JIA, which includes several types of arthritis previously known as juvenile rheumatoid arthritis, may over time include a variety of symptoms, such as muscle and soft tissue tightening, bone erosion, joint misalignment and changes in growth patterns.

In addition to watching for symptoms for at least six weeks, the number six also figures prominently in another part of the diagnostic process. To identify the specific type of JIA, your child's doctor will wait to see how her symptoms unfold during the first six months after onset. As with the previous JRA criteria, the number of joints affected during those first six months remains significant. In addition, the JIA criteria also rely on other results, such as those from the rheumatoid factor blood test, to help further categorize patients.

Based on her symptoms, your child may be diagnosed with one of the following categories of JIA:

OLIGOARTHRITIS: This type, formerly known as pauciarticular, is diagnosed when four or fewer joints — "pauci" and "oligo" mean "few" — are involved within the first six months. It's particularly common in Caucasian children. The diagnosis accounts for about 60 percent of all new JIA diagnoses. Girls are more likely to be diagnosed with oligoarthritis and to experience eye inflammation, a disease called uveitis. Oligoarthritis typically develops by age 6. At diagnosis, only one joint is involved in about half of the cases and it's commonly a joint in the leg, such as the knee or the ankle.

If your child also tests positive for a particular antibody in the blood, called the antinuclear antibody (ANA), she faces the greatest risk of developing eye inflammation and will be monitored very closely for eye problems. Compared with other types of JIA, children with oligoarthritis are less vulnerable to severe joint functioning problems.

Under the JIA criteria, oligoarthritis is broken into two groups. Children in which the arthritis is confined to four or fewer limbs fall into a category called persistent oligoarthritis. Some children will go on to later develop (after the six-month window) symptoms in additional limbs and will be diagnosed with extended oligoarthritis.

POLYARTHRITIS: This type of JIA — "poly" means "many" — is diagnosed when five or more joints are involved during the first six months. Roughly 25 percent of children with JIA have polyarthritis. Like oligoarthritis, it's more common in girls, but its onset can occur any time in childhood. Both large and small joints, such as the fingers and toes, may be involved. Your child also may experience arthritis in the neck or the jaw, making chewing and opening her mouth more difficult.

Unlike oligoarthritis, polyarthritis more frequently affects joints on both sides of the body, such as the right and the left knees. Children with polyarthritis might face a lower risk of eye inflammation, but will still need

---

JUVENILE IDIOPATHIC ARTHRITIS: SYMPTOMS

Some typical symptoms include:

- Joint swelling
- Limping, or change in walking
- Persistent fever
- Reduced activity
- Reluctance to use an arm or a leg
- Stiffness when waking up
- Change of interest in activities

to see an ophthalmologist on a regular basis, as the risk of possible eye problems is still there.

The JIA criteria also subdivides children with polyarthritis into two categories, those who test positive for rheumatoid factor (RF) — an antibody found in the blood — and those who don't. The RF-positive form of the disease usually emerges in the elementary school years or later. It's

....

JIA vs. JRA – UNDERSTANDING THE DIFFERENCE

Juvenile idiopathic arthritis and juvenile rheumatoid arthritis can't be used interchangeably, as there are differences between the diagnoses they include. For more detail about the new JIA language that's being adopted, you might want to refer to this chart:

NEW CLASSIFICATION	DESCRIPTION	OLD CLASSIFICATION
Systemic Arthritis	Affects the entire body, not just joints and is preceded by a fever and a faint rash; typically diagnosed in young children	Systemic-onset JRA
Oligoarthritis	Arthritis of one to four joints during the first six months of disease; typically diagnosed in young children	Pauciarticular JRA
Persistent	Affects no more than four joints after first six months	
Extended	Affects more than four joints after first six months	
Polyarthritis (RF-negative)	Affects five or more joints in the first six months of disease; test for rheumatoid factor (RF) are negative	Polyarticular JRA (RF does not alter classification)
Polyarthritis (RF-positive)	Affects five or more joints in the first six months of disease; tests for RF are positive on two occasions at least two months apart; usually appears in late childhood	Polyarticular JRA (RF does not alter classification)
Enthesitis-related Arthritis	Affects the entheses — where tendons attach to bone — and can move to the spine or develop as one of the juvenile spondyloarthropathies; affects boys more often than girls	Excluded in JRA classification, but some youth in this group at onset may be similar to late-onset pauciarticular JRA
Psoriatic Arthritis	Arthritis that is preceded or follows development of the skin condition psoriasis; pitting or ridging of fingernails also a sign	Excluded in JRA classification
Other	Arthritis of unknown cause persisting for at least six weeks that either does not fulfill criteria for any categories or fulfills criteria for more than one category	

MANAGING SYSTEMIC ARTHRITIS
Taylor Six's Story

The fever would come and go, but Taylor Six couldn't quite shake it. When her mother, Pam, first took her to the doctor, the pediatrician suggested she was suffering from a virus or the flu. Just wait it out, he suggested.

So they tried. Over the next several weeks, the 8-year-old girl missed 14 days of school while her symptoms came and went and changed in ways that perplexed her teachers and family. Sometimes she'd feel better in the morning with no fever and relatively little discomfort. Then her temperature and pain would spike after lunch and the school nurse would send her home. Or, she'd awaken feeling miserable only to watch the symptoms mysteriously lift later in the day. "You think you have this kid who is messing with your mind and is trying to get out of school," her mother says.

Increasingly, though, Pam worried. The prior year, Taylor developed a similar fever and flu-like symptoms. Her pediatrician had raised the possibility of arthritis, but by the time Taylor saw a rheumatologist several weeks later, she felt fine.

This time, after Taylor's bouts of fever, her regular pediatrician ran some blood tests and then got on the phone with Cincinnati Children's Hospital Medical Center. The next day Taylor and her mother made the first of many trips, nearly two hours each way from their Kentucky home.

For several years afterward, Taylor enjoyed long periods without symptoms, marred only by annual flares. The resurgence of symptoms seemed to follow a pattern, occurring between January and May and persisting at least a couple of weeks. During flares, she would take as many as 14 pills a day. Some nights, the mother-daughter pair would spend the wee hours in the bathroom, Taylor soaking in the tub in search of relief.

Then her flares became more frequent and more extended. She now takes a biologic agent, which seems, at least initially, to ease her pain and other symptoms. Most importantly, the active 12-year-old — a softball player when her symptoms allow — is feeling better.

> "She'd awaken feeling miserable only to watch the symptoms mysteriously lift later in the day."

the type most similar to adult rheumatoid arthritis, with symptoms such as rheumatoid nodules. Children with RF-positive polyarthritis are more vulnerable to severe disease and related joint erosion than those who test negative for rheumatoid factor.

SYSTEMIC: Involving about 10 percent of JIA cases, systemic arthritis affects the entire body, not just the joints. Both boys and girls are equally vulnerable to systemic arthritis. Although the symptoms can start at any time during childhood, they generally emerge before or during the elementary school years.

The first sign might be a stubborn fever, sometimes appearing weeks or months before your child complains of any joint discomfort or mobility issues. The fever can be quite high, appearing once or twice daily, before returning to normal. By all indications, your child might seem fine after the fever but before joint symptoms appear. Fevers also may be accompanied by a faint rash, which ebbs and flares over the course of days. Often described as pinkish or salmon-colored, it's not contagious.

Since this illness can affect the entire body, inflammation may occur elsewhere, such as enlarging the spleen or irritating the coverings of the lungs or heart. In many cases, the fever and other systemic symptoms will fade over time.

Eye inflammation is not common, but your child's vision will still need to be checked regularly.

Potentially, the disease can influence your child's growth and appetite, making good nutrition a high priority. But the course of the disease, including the number of joints involved, can be highly variable and individual. Only over time will your child's doctor have a better sense of the challenges she faces.

ENTHESITIS-RELATED: This type, which wasn't included under the original JRA criteria, involves inflammation of the entheses, the places where tendons attach to the bone. Boys are more often diagnosed with this condition. The arthritis can be mild, involving four or fewer joints in roughly half of cases. In some children, arthritis can move to the spine. Frequently, they test positive for the HLA-B27 gene.

Over time, your child may develop one of the various conditions also known as juvenile spondyloarthropathies, which may, but do not necessarily, affect the spine. Some of those diseases include: juvenile ankylosing spondylitis, arthritis associated with inflammatory bowel disease and reactive arthritis.

JUVENILE PSORIATIC ARTHRITIS: In this form of arthritis, the skin condition called psoriasis may precede or follow arthritis symptoms, sometimes by years. The rash may appear as scaly red blotches, emerging behind the ears or on the eye lids, elbows, knees or scalp. Your child may have a family history of psoriasis. Another common sign: a pitting or unusual ridging on the fingernails.

OTHER: Any arthritis of unknown cause, with symptoms continuing at least six weeks, that doesn't meet criteria for any one type of JIA or involves symptoms that span two or more types.

Beyond JIA

Along with juvenile idiopathic arthritis, pediatric rheumatologists treat many other conditions in which arthritis is either the primary component or a symptom of the underlying disease.

JUVENILE DERMATOMYOSITIS: An inflammatory disease, juvenile dermatomyositis causes muscle weakness and a skin rash on the eyelids and knuckles. Roughly one in five affected children also have arthritis, but it's likely to be mild. The disease can result in muscle weakness in the trunk, shoulders and upper legs that potentially limits running, climbing stairs and other activities.

JUVENILE LUPUS: Lupus is a disease of the immune system; the most common form is systemic lupus erythematosus, or SLE. Adults are diagnosed more often than children and the disease is far more common in women. Lupus can affect the joints, skin, kidneys, blood and other areas of the body. Symptoms may include a butterfly-shaped rash that bridges the nose and the cheeks, a scaly-type rash on the face or neck, sensitivity to sunlight, pain in the joints and chest pain.

JUVENILE SCLERODERMA: Scleroderma, which literally means "hard skin," describes a group of conditions that causes the skin to tighten and harden. There are two basic forms, one of which affects the entire body, and one that is localized — primarily a skin disease — and occurs more commonly in children. The skin may become either thickened or thinned, lighter or darker, but is often smooth or shiny in appearance. The skin changes for localized disease can occur anywhere, from the face to the arms and legs, or on the trunk. The more widespread, systemic form, which affects internal organs, tends to affect the skin of the fingers, hands, forearms and face, and is more frequently is seen in girls.

KAWASAKI DISEASE: First described by Japanese pediatrician Tomisaku Kawasaki, who noticed common patterns in a group of children — inflammatory-type symptoms followed in later years by heart complications. The disease, which primarily affects infants and young children, frequently starts with a high fever. Other changes may include a visible rash or a swelling or redness around the hands or feet, followed a few weeks later by peeling around the fingers and toes. Although arthritis can occur, the most serious concern is the inflammation of the blood vessels themselves; careful monitoring for heart complications is necessary.

MIXED CONNECTIVE TISSUE DISEASE: This disease may include features of arthritis, lupus, dermatomyositis and scleroderma, and is associated with very high levels of a particular antinuclear antibody (anti-RNP).

Of course, there are a number of other noninflammatory causes of pain and stiffness, sometimes chronic, in children.

NONINFLAMMATORY RHEUMATIC CONDITIONS:

• **Fibromyalgia:** This chronic pain syndrome can cause stiffness and aching, fatigue, disrupted sleep and other symptoms. More common in girls, fibromyalgia is seldom diagnosed before puberty. It is not a form of arthritis but is a related condition that is often treated by a rheumatologist.

• **Growing Pains:** The cause unknown, growing pains typically occur in the evening or during the night, but don't cause morning stiffness like arthritis does. Symptoms are not focused on the joints, but rather include deep aching or cramping pains in the thigh or calf, or sometimes the arms. Girls and boys are equally affected.

In the years ahead, arthritis terms may again change, as researchers become more sophisticated in unraveling genetic differences between different types of the disease. In the meantime, if you educate yourself about your child's diagnosis, including long-term risk factors, you'll be better equipped to discuss and weigh treatment options with your child's medical team. ●

CHAPTER THREE

How Does Juvenile Arthritis Develop?

"What caused this illness in my child?" Pediatric rheumatologists get this question all too often, and may have little to offer in response. For researchers, too, the mysteries stack up. What combination of forces launches the inflammatory cascade that results in symptoms? Why are girls frequently more vulnerable than boys? And what might account for the elevated risk in certain groups, such as Native Americans?

Although much has been learned about joints and inflammation, at this point researchers have identified far more questions than answers. But they have made some progress in recent years. This includes taking initial steps toward unraveling the complex interplay between genes and environmental factors that are believed to foster the emergence of autoimmune diseases like juvenile arthritis.

Autoimmune diseases are so called because they develop when something goes awry in the body's natural immune system. "Auto" means self. Instead of protecting the body against external onslaughts, such as flu viruses, the cells of the immune system become the body's own worst enemy, attacking its own cells by mistake. In juvenile arthritis, the result can be painful inflammation, fever and other symptoms. But juvenile arthritis is only one of many autoimmune diseases; others include multiple sclerosis, Type 1 diabetes and some thyroid disorders.

By all indications, the genetic links are complex. Unlike diseases associated with a single gene, such as cystic fibrosis or sickle cell anemia, juvenile arthritis is believed to be associated with a number of genes. To date, at least a dozen genes — out of an estimated 20,000 to 40,000 in the entire human genome — have been identified as strongly associated with juvenile idiopathic arthritis (JIA) specifically. In addition, several hundred genes are considered to be candidate genes. They are under scrutiny because it is believed they potentially play a role by expressing themselves differently in patients with the common form of JIA.

Pinning JIA to a genetic cause is difficult because the condition rarely runs in families. If your child develops Type 1 diabetes, for example, the likelihood that a sibling also will be diagnosed is significantly greater than if she develops a type of JIA. A national registry housed at Cincinnati Children's Hospital Medical Center has been striving to locate pairs of siblings, both diagnosed with a type of JIA, to collect genetic and other family information. Sponsored by the National Institutes of Health, the initiative is called the JRA Affected Sib-Pair Registry. By early 2008, researchers had enrolled about 220 sibling pairs; they estimate that roughly 300 sibling pairs in all live in the United States.

The familial connection between types of JIA and the broader category of autoimmune diseases appears to be stronger, according to other findings by Cincinnati Children's researchers. By sifting through data in the sibling-pair registry, they've determined that close relatives (parents, siblings, aunts, uncles) of children with juvenile arthritis are three times more likely to be diagnosed with some type of autoimmune disease.

Autoimmune Disease: Trunk and Branches

One way to understand the relationship between autoimmunity and specific diagnoses is to picture a tree trunk and its branches. The trunk represents the broader category of autoimmunity, those genes that boost your child's vulnerability to developing any one of a number of autoimmune diseases. Branching from that broader susceptibility are a number of other genes and genetic markers that contribute to specific diseases, such as ankylosing spondylitis, systemic lupus erythematosus (SLE) or Type 1 diabetes.

RHEUMATIC DISEASES:
ETHNIC DIFFERENCES AND NATIVE AMERICANS

To date, most of the research about rates of childhood rheumatic disease has focused on Caucasian populations in Europe and North America. Several recent studies, though, indicate that Native American children face a greater risk of certain types of arthritis, a higher rate that — if better understood — might provide insights helpful to children of all backgrounds.

In one of the studies which included two Native American health service regions in the United States, researchers identified a considerably higher prevalence of juvenile rheumatoid arthritis among children of the northern plains tribes, mainly in Montana and Wyoming. They discovered that this group had a rate of 115 cases per 100,000 people, about 10 times that reported in Europe in recent studies. In comparison, Native American children studied in Oklahoma had similar rates of JRA to kids in Europe.

Researchers at the University of Oklahoma College of Medicine theorized that people from the northern plains tribes might be particularly susceptible to juvenile arthritis compared with other Native American populations. They also considered that this group may comprise more children with full-blooded, rather than mixed, Indian ancestry.

Polyarticular juvenile rheumatoid arthritis or spondyloarthropathy were the two most common diagnoses. Virtually no cases of oligoarticular (pauciarticular) JRA were identified, a pattern that's appeared elsewhere. While oligoarticular arthritis is the most common diagnosis in Caucasian children, it's far less common in children of some other backgrounds, based on studies of children in Asia, South Africa and African-American children in Detroit.

Still, as the 2004 study reveals, the Native American tribes have diverse heritages and thus their relative arthritis risk shouldn't be lumped together. Those differences do, however, offer opportunities for researchers trying to unravel the genetic underpinnings of different rheumatic diseases, says James N. Jarvis, MD, a study author and chief of pediatric rheumatology at the University of Oklahoma College of Medicine.

Dr. Jarvis offers the Oklahoma Choctaw as one illustrative example. One study, he writes, has shown a very high prevalence of systemic sclerosis — a form of scleroderma — in Choctaw people living in Oklahoma, but not Mississippi.

This difference in prevalence, he points out, may be attributable to a single pedigree, descended from a common founder who lived in Mississippi before the group was forced to relocate. Digging further might result in potentially powerful genetic insights.

Researchers interested in autoimmunity are looking into the HLA (human leukocyte antigen) complex to learn more about what may cause JIA. This cluster of genes, which reside on chromosome 6, is believed to play a significant role in fighting infection, as well as in the development of autoimmunity. In addition to the genes themselves, there are also related proteins that help the body's immune system distinguish between its own cells and nasty invaders such as viruses.

We're still in the early days of understanding what genetic markers may mean for our health, but researchers are starting to associate certain genes on the HLA complex with an increased risk of specific diagnoses. Testing positive for HLA-B27, as has been previously discussed on page 9, is associated with a higher risk of developing one of the spondyloarthropathies. Other genes, such as HLA-DR1 and HLA-DR4, appear to be linked with children who have rheumatoid factor-positive polyarthritis.

HLA isn't the only autoimmune region under the genetic microscope. In recent years, researchers have turned their sights on the PTPN22 variation, located on another chromosome, which they believe is associated with adult rheumatoid arthritis, juvenile rheumatoid arthritis, lupus and autoimmune thyroid disease.

So what does this new knowledge mean for you? Important genetic tests are being developed now, but their results may still not tell us what we need to know. Insightful in some cases, they may only provide a piece of the puzzle. Take the HLA-B27 test: The overwhelming majority of those diagnosed with ankylosing spondylitis, an arthritis that primarily affects the spine, will test positive for HLA-B27, particularly if they are Caucasian. But individuals can carry HLA-B27 without developing any related arthritis of the spine.

By the same token, genes aren't singularly bad. For every gene or genetic marker, such as a protein, that might nudge your child a little closer to developing an autoimmune condition, there are believed to be another set of genetic components that step in to slow or halt the process.

Furthermore, genes are likely only part of a two-step process. As with many other diseases, such as cancer, environmental triggers are believed to play a role. Your child may, to a greater or lesser degree, have a genetic profile that boosts her risk of developing arthritis, but having a particular genetic makeup, when coupled with certain outside influences, may tip the balance.

These environmental influences are still unknown; the role of infections is only one of a number of possibilities being studied. For example, there's no conclusive evidence, to date, that a pregnant woman's nutrition or other habits during pregnancy contribute to a child's arthritis, so delete that fear from your list of worries.

Applying Genetic Advances

This alphabet soup of genetic markers may become more relevant to your child's life sooner than you might think.

By identifying and better understanding the roles of specific genes and related markers, researchers will start applying that knowledge in a number of ways. They may be able to more quickly isolate your child's type of arthritis, which will help dictate treatment choices. At the same time, they may pick up genetic clues that help them predict the long-term course of her disease. Medication treatment also will one day benefit, thanks to an exciting technique called gene expression profiling.

Researchers now believe that genes alone do not dictate your child's response to a particular drug. There's another crucial component: How do your genes turn on and off in response to that drug? By studying the response — or expression — of those genes to specific medications, researchers can learn more about which types of juvenile arthritis respond to which treatments. Unlike clinical trials, which essentially use a trial-and-error approach to determine how and when drugs work best, genetic expression profiling could one day help your child's doctor better tailor the medication regimen to her genetic strain of disease.

Less time wasted in trying medications will reduce both cost and frustration. Most importantly, it will cut short the time required to get your child's inflammation under control. Hopefully, the result will be less daily discomfort and the derailing of some of the longer-term effects of the disease. ●

CHAPTER FOUR

Managing Your Child's Medical Care

Your child's diagnosis may seem overwhelming at first, both logistically and emotionally. Even when her disease is well controlled, you'll be busy tracking down laboratory results, filling out insurance forms and juggling doctors' appointments — along with work and home responsibilities.

Don't despair! To help your child stay pain-free and functioning well, you'll have far more than your child's pediatric rheumatologist on which to rely. In a given year, your child may also visit an eye doctor for checkups, an occupational or physical therapist to promote body flexibility and perhaps a social worker or psychologist. You'll also discover that other clinicians, such as a nurse or the corner pharmacist, will become key resources — and champions — in keeping your child healthy.

To help keep all of those balls in the air, though, you'll need to employ good communication, disciplined organization and, on some days, a sense of humor. Internet research, e-mail communication and other technological tools may provide some short cuts. Also, don't hesitate — in fact, you should insist — to involve your child. The sooner your child understands her own medical care, whether it's asking the doctor a question or filling out a medication chart, the sooner she'll be able to manage her own illness.

Getting the Most From Your Child's Medical Visits

Given the sometimes compressed nature of today's doctor visits, it's important to maximize your time, particularly if you'd like to discuss several issues. Regardless of whether this is your child's first visit to a particular physician or it's an ongoing relationship, there are several ways you can prepare.

BEFORE THE VISIT: You might schedule your child for blood work and other diagnostic tests before the appointment, if she's already a patient. That way, your doctor will have time to review the results and discuss them in person. If it's your first visit, call ahead to make sure that your child's medical records have been sent by the prior physician's office.

If it would be beneficial, ask a friend or family member to come along. Perhaps that individual would make your child more comfortable, as well as help you recall crucial information. Alternatively, ask whether it's OK to use a tape recorder or to get a copy of the clinic's note, so that you don't lose track of important details.

Prepare ahead of time. Jot down information to tell the doctor or questions that you'd like to ask. Sit down, ideally with your child, and prepare a progress report. Among the questions the doctor might ask: "Have you been following your treatment plan? How have you been feeling?" Discuss these questions with your child. Also, ask your child to rate her pain. Not just on a 1-to-10 scale, but also ask her to describe it. Does it feel more like a numbing pain, for example, or a stabbing pain?

Make sure you know the dosages of your child's medications, along with their names. Include over-the-counter and prescription medication. You might want to bring the pill bottles along, particularly if your child is seeing other physician specialists, such as a gastroenterologist, along with her pediatric rheumatologist. If refills are required, add that request to your list of questions.

DURING THE VISIT: When you sit down with your child's doctor, begin with your most important concerns first. Encourage your child to participate, not only by answering the doctor's questions, but also sharing any issues that she might have.

Besides updating the doctor about your child's most significant symptoms, be sure to also discuss how your child is functioning in normal activities, and how the treatments she is using aligns with your child's daily routine. For example, is the medication effective enough to allow your child to participate in dance, soccer and other activities that she values? How about the medication schedule? If taking medication four times a day is difficult for your child, the doctor might be able to prescribe medication twice daily. Don't be afraid to speak up and ask for a modified approach that you think will work better for your child.

You might want to take some notes as the doctor talks, so you don't forget a detail later. If your child's doctor suggests a new treatment, don't be shy about questioning why. Be sure to get a sense of the timeline. When will it be clear if the new medication, exercise or other approach is working? If you and your child both understand what the treatments will do to help her, your child may be more willing to stick to the treatment plan over the long haul. Remember: Arthritis is not a disease that gets better with a single shot or pill. It's a chronic condition that can only improve with a commitment to sticking to a long-term plan of taking medications, exercise, eating right and more.

And, don't shy away from asking your child's doctor to explain or clarify some medical details or jargon; your child would benefit from the additional explanation. When unsure, try repeating back your understanding of the directions. Request written materials that you may review later, or a nurse you can consult with, in case you have any follow-up questions.

DON'T BE AFRAID TO:

- Tell the doctor that you're not happy about your child's treatment progress.
- Request details about treatment options or suggest a change in your child's treatment.
- Find out how much a particular medication costs, or if there are generic options.
- Negotiate with your doctor, if there's a particular activity your child really wants to do. Perhaps with an accommodation, or a change in medication approach, it might be feasible.

Doctors are often busy and visits can seem all too short or even rushed. Make sure your child's appointment or discussion with the doctor isn't all about blood work results, medication side effects and other clinical details.

BETWEEN APPOINTMENTS

Before you leave the doctor's office, check how the physician and his staff handle a variety of issues that might crop up — from a prescription holdup to an emergency crisis:

- How does your doctor define an emergency — and what should you do?
- How are routine questions handled? Is e-mail an option?
- What's the turnaround time to get a question answered?
- How are prescription refills handled?

PERSONAL ESSAY

A CRASH COURSE IN ARTHRITIS
Jeanne McQuade's Essay

When my daughter, Holland, was diagnosed with juvenile rheumatoid arthritis shortly before the age of 2, I was scared, upset and confused. I was angry because I felt I had absolutely no control over what was happening to my daughter. The only way I felt in control was to learn all I could.

Early on, I started a journal to log every doctor's visit, every medication and the results. I researched every drug she was prescribed before I would let her take it and logged it in my journal, along with any side effects I saw. I kept this journal faithfully for two years. After awhile, the information became too much and I was unable to log every single thing. But, if asked, I would be able to recite every medication, every side effect, everything that has happened to my daughter in the past 13 years.

I learned, with the help of a friend in nursing school, how to decipher the PDR (*Physician's Desk Reference*), and other medical books. I learned from medical assistants how to get my 3-year-old to swallow pills, which she did like a pro. I also gave seminars at Holland's schools, when she was younger, to inform the teachers and students about her disease. Every year, I ask the doctor to write a letter stating the details of her disease as well as upcoming appointments and how often she needs to go. This has been very handy for us regarding excused absences.

In the past four years, I took two medical classes, a medical terminology class and an anatomy class so I could better understand what the doctors were saying and what was going on inside my daughter's body.

I like to think that I'm well-versed in the areas of gastroenterology, ophthalmology, rheumatology and the skeletal system. As I said, this disease made me angry and the only way I could channel this anger was to talk and read. Lots of reading.

At the time of this writing, after a five-month flare, Holland is finally under control with the right medication and an understanding doctor. My daughter is a fighter. But sometimes, when I am alone, I cannot help but think about what it must be like to start a life with arthritis. And to never know a life, thus far, without pain.

—*Jeanne McQuade lives near Detroit.*

> "The only way I felt in control was to learn all I could."

Your child's questions and concerns also should be asked and answered. Take time to celebrate the successes, whether it's a recent basketball trophy or even the fact that she can now tie her shoes without help each morning. No matter what her age, this appointment is ultimately about your child.

AFTER THE VISIT: To remain on track, get your child involved in her own treatment plan. Brainstorm with her about the best times of day to exercise and the optimal location. Develop other strategies to help keep joint health front and center. For example, a medication chart could be designed and hung on the bathroom mirror or the refrigerator, so it's easily visible.

Don't alter your child's treatment plan without consultation with your health-care professional. If the rhythm of your child's day makes certain elements of exercise or other treatment difficult, call your doctor's office to discuss alternatives. Above all, don't allow your child to stop taking medication because symptoms appear to be fading, or because she thinks the drugs aren't working. Some medications can take time, potentially months, to pay off in relief. Consistency is crucial.

Neither should your child start any over-the-counter medication without contacting the doctor's office first. The risks are two-fold. The medication on the drug store or natural food store shelf may be wasted money, with no benefit. Even worse, they could undercut or interact dangerously with the powerful drugs that she's already taking.

Between appointments, don't rely on your memory — or your child's for that matter — to track ongoing or emerging symptoms or functioning difficulties. It might be helpful for you or your child to jot down side effects, exercise challenges and other issues that crop up (on a simple monthly calendar, for example) so you're prepared for the next appointment.

Finding the Right Doctor

Sometimes the chemistry just doesn't work between you, your child and the doctor. You might discover that your child's doctor doesn't communicate well with you or your child. Or, you're losing sleep that your child's arthritis hasn't been adequately controlled.

With arthritis specialists in such short supply, you might be reluctant to shop around. Try some intervention strategies first. Consider your own interactions. Are you being specific in the questions you ask? Are you reluctant to speak up? It's OK to rephrase a question or request additional explanation if you feel like your doctor hasn't addressed your concerns or your child's questions.

Still not satisfied? Before looking elsewhere, talk with your doctor. Approach the conversation like a negotiation, one that's handled in a collaborative, non-confrontational way. Don't just express your gripes — present solutions as well. After all, you're both on the same team, fighting for the best treatment picture — now and in the future — for your child. Some families find it helpful to talk with the team nurse or social worker about their concerns and possible solutions.

If you're worried about your child's mobility, pain or other symptoms, you might want to request a second opinion or consultation. One approach, if you live a long distance from a pediatric rheumatologist, is to take a one-time or once-a-year trip to gain some outside perspective. Once you locate the specialist you want to consult, ask your child's current doctor for a referral. Don't be afraid to make that request; a good physician shouldn't feel threatened by it.

Besides, consulting with an outside specialist doesn't preclude your child from continuing with her regular doctor. In situations where travel is difficult, you might decide to use the regular doctor for most appointments, but the long-distance specialist can be available for consultation and questions.

Staying Organized

As you've no doubt learned, you could quickly become overwhelmed by the massive paperwork required to document and stay abreast of your child's illness. Besides her medical records, you also will stockpile numerous other forms: laboratory results, immunization records, prescriptions, school documents and so on.

Or at least you should be stockpiling those records. Despite the headaches involved, keep a complete record of your child's treatment if your family moves or

....

BEYOND DIAGNOSIS — QUESTIONS TO ASK

After your child's arthritis is diagnosed, you might have more questions than answers. As you meet with your child's doctor and other clinicians, here are some areas you might want to explore with them:

- What's the purpose of this treatment?
- How and when will this treatment make my child feel better?
- What potential side effects should I watch for?
- What symptoms warrant a call to the doctor?
- What are the medication alternatives?
- What other health professionals should my child see?
- What lifestyle changes should we consider?
- What assistive devices could help my child accomplish daily tasks?
- What school or home accommodations should we consider?
- How do you think my child's arthritis will progress in the future?
- Are there any local programs designed for children with arthritis?

your child adds a new doctor. Although medical records can be sent between physicians' offices, you might be able to pull from your own records more quickly to verify a side effect or how long your child took a particular drug. Over time, your stash of documents also may include details related to your child's other activities, such as a medical release form to participate in a sport or documentation of her school absences.

Some parents will purchase a binder specifically to track the various issues — medical and otherwise — relevant to their child's arthritis diagnosis. By using a three-ring binder, you'll have plenty of space to add documents and dividers to keep everything straight. Another organizational trick: Invest in some clear plastic pockets to store smaller items, such as prescriptions or business cards.

Everyone's approach is different, but here are some strategies to consider

....

INTERNET RESEARCH AND E-MAIL: PROS AND CONS

The Internet can offer a wealth of medical information. Nearly nine out of every 10 Americans with a chronic condition have gone online to research a health topic, according to a 2006 survey conducted by the Pew Internet & American Life Project. Slightly more than two-thirds of those e-patients, as they're sometimes called, use what they learn online to question their doctor in more detail or to request a second opinion.

That doesn't mean that everyone is a fan of virtual information and communication. Doctors have been slower to adopt e-mail communication, because of concerns about protecting patient privacy. And, if they do, the exchanges will probably be restricted to sharing lab results or answering a quick question.

Still, with a little virtual savvy, the Internet can provide a rich resource for yourself and your child. Some tools and potential pitfalls to keep in mind:

Consider (and Narrow) the Source: If you type "juvenile" and "arthritis" into a general search engine like Google, about 500,000 responses will appear on your computer screen. Before you give the information any credence, check out the source. Who is the site's sponsor? How often is the site updated? (Usually a date at the end will let you know how fresh the information is.) A safer bet, at least initially, would be to start with sites affiliated with medical professionals or organizations, such as the Arthritis Foundation (www. arthritis.org) or the American

College of Rheumatology (www.rheumatology.org).

Consult Your Doctor: Don't read — or react — to what you see online in a vacuum. Bring in the studies or other information that interests or concerns you. Doctors are becoming more accustomed to patients, or their parents, walking in with a sheaf of paper in hand. And, of course, consult with a medical practitioner before trying an alternative remedy, exercise or other treatment touted online.

Avoid Pitfalls: Avoid sites that offer outlandish claims or require you to pay a fee to obtain information. Double check your spelling if your typing turns up an odd-looking list of references. Also, pinpoint your search criteria so you don't unearth a flood of useless results.

as you attempt to rein in your snowballing paperwork:

- **Don't Fly Solo:** One parent shouldn't be left to do all of the organizing. By getting other family members involved, it will be easier to stay on top of this. If your child is old enough, get her involved. To prevent the task from taking over, try to file accumulating paperwork at least once a week.

- **Copies, etc.:** Keep several copies of your child's medical records on hand so you don't have to return to the doctor's office every time they are requested. Physician offices frequently charge for copies. Some laboratory facilities may not keep X-rays and other images indefinitely, so request a copy from them.

- **Safer Storage:** One option is to store a copy in a fire safe. Another is to start a backup master file with a friend or family member. If your child spends a lot of time at someone else's house, you can give them a medical emergency permission form in case a crisis arises.

- **What to Keep:** Among some of the paperwork doctors and parents recommend that you keep include:
  - Notes from your child's medical team, including physical and occupational therapy reports.
  - Laboratory results, including blood work and diagnostic images.
  - List of medications, including prescriptions and over-the-counter.
  - A medication history, outlining past medications, dates and any side effects, in the event that your child changes doctors.
  - Surgical records.
  - Insurance information, including claims.
  - A record of school absences, in case a dispute arises later regarding how much time your child has missed.
  - A running list of questions ready for the next doctor's visit.

Step by Step

Some days the medical logistics might seem overwhelming, particularly if your child's symptoms are resurging. Try not to look too far ahead, but instead focus on the doctor you need to contact that week or those insurance questions you need to resolve most urgently. Don't be afraid to lean on friends and family members for all types of help. Battling a long-term illness like juvenile arthritis can feel like a marathon, but one that can be tackled step by step, relying on your medical team and your own personal safety net. ●

....

CHAPTER FIVE

Treatment Goals and Remission

Many days, effective treatment — and thus relief — may seem like an elusive target, seemingly on the horizon and then moving just out of reach. Thwarting your child's complex autoimmune disease is no small challenge, one which may require several prescriptions, along with exercise and other medical interventions. It may also require several bouts of trial and error with different medications and doses before you find one that's "just right." But pediatric rheumatologists are increasingly optimistic.

The ongoing advances in medication are reframing treatment goals. Instead of just trying to ease your child's symptoms, it's more feasible than ever before to substantially minimize them or, ideally, eliminate them entirely for a period of time. The goal is to identify the right drug, or combination of drugs, that enables your child to enjoy all of her favorite activities, whether that's ballet, painting or tearing up the soccer field.

Then there's that wonderful word — remission — in which the disease becomes inactive, at least temporarily. What counts as remission? Leading researchers still grapple with the exact criteria. They're engaged in ongoing research that hopefully will unearth better data regarding your child's chance of remission.

Understanding Remission

Remissions can occur spontaneously, for reasons that are unclear, with symptoms disappearing for months to years. Those spontaneous remissions helped spawn the myth that children simply grow out of their arthritis by adulthood. In fact, researchers now believe many of those children suffered symptoms down the road, after they "graduated" from seeing their pediatric specialists.

Researchers also believe that medication treatment can promote remission in some children. It's unclear exactly how this happens, and no blood tests can confirm disease remission. But it's believed that the drug intervention helps derail the inflammatory cascade of symptoms in some way, perhaps by resetting or rebooting the immune system.

Thus, as new classes of medication have been discovered, a wonderful dilemma has developed: How do we define remission?

It's not an easy task, as it turns out. Until recently, the term "remission" had variable interpretations, even among researchers. A review of 24 papers published about juvenile rheumatoid arthritis in 2000 and 2001 identified only three that used the same definition of remission. Researchers had to find common ground. Without standardized criteria, it would be difficult to weigh the relative long-term results of various medication regimens.

In 2003, a consensus conference was held, attended by pediatric rheumatologists from nine countries and several research groups, including the Childhood Arthritis and Rheumatology Research Alliance (CARRA). By sifting through data and feedback from 130 pediatric rheumatologists describing how they define inactive disease, the conference members hammered out criteria for several types of juvenile idiopathic arthritis.

Criteria for Remission

The conference yielded rules that physicians could easily use in their offices, along with a time table to follow, to assess whether your child is in remission. Remission was broken into several phases, beginning with the criteria for inactive disease, followed by the time tables for diagnosing remission both on and off medication.

CRITERIA FOR INACTIVE DISEASE:

• No joints with active arthritis.

PERSONAL STORY

WAITING FOR THE NEXT FLARE
Victoria Mischley's Story

It was a magical summer month, as long as it lasted. Victoria Mischley had been off her dreaded methotrexate for four months and was taking only etanercept (*Enbrel*) and an NSAID (nonsteroidal anti-inflammatory drug). At a doctor's visit, Victoria's pediatric rheumatologist reported no signs of active arthritis. For the first time since her diagnosis with polyarthritis two years previously, Victoria could begin the countdown, marking off the months toward remission and weaning off the drugs entirely.

"A month — that's all the time I had to live that little happy fantasy [of potential remission]," says her mom, Michelle.

Then, a month later, the 8-year-old woke up, complaining of pain in her ankles. Over the years, Michelle has become painfully sensitized to the sometimes subtle signals that Victoria's disease is flaring. Victoria might start awaking for no apparent reason in the night. Or, during the day, she might be a little more emotional, a little grumpier.

But the biggest shock of any flare — and that summer flare in particular — is what it symbolizes,

> "I wasn't prepared for what it feels like to go through a flare."

says Michelle, a Michigan mother of three.

"I wasn't prepared for what it feels like to go through a flare — the disappointment. You think the whole shock of your child having arthritis is hard. It's almost as hard knowing that your child is flaring again."

Over the next three years, Victoria's medication regimen swelled until she was taking large amounts of a variety of drugs. Most days, Victoria is determined not to let her discomfort slow her down. "If she's around her friends, she'll do anything they do, even if it kills her," her mother says.

But she battles a particularly stubborn case of polyarthritis, as Victoria's doctor acknowledged at a recent appointment. Driving the two hours home afterward, Michelle called her mother from her cell phone. She couldn't help tearing up as they talked, even though Victoria sat just a few feet away.

"You want to be positive — you want to be the perfect mom," she says, adding, "I really think she's going to have this to some degree for her whole life."

- No fever, rash, serositis (inflammation of the tissues lining the lungs, heart, abdomen or organs within), no enlargement of the spleen or lymph nodes that can be attributed to juvenile arthritis.
- No active uveitis, or inflammation of the eye.
- Normal C-reactive proteins and erythrocyte sedimentation rate (ESR).
- No disease activity indicated on the physician's global assessment of disease activity.

CRITERIA FOR CLINICAL REMISSION ON MEDICATION:

- The criteria for inactive disease above must be met for a minimum of six continuous months while the patient is taking medication.

CRITERIA FOR CLINICAL REMISSION OFF MEDICATION:

- The criteria for inactive disease must be met for a minimum of 12 continuous months while off all arthritis medications.

These remission criteria, it should be noted, are considered preliminary, subject to change as researchers fine tune their understanding of juvenile arthritis. Several uncertainties continue to complicate the remission question. One is smoldering disease. Although your child may be classified as

....

FLARES: PREVENTION AND INTERVENTIONS

Stay on top of your child's medication — that's the best way to prevent a flare. Your child may be old enough to take charge of her own pills or injections, but still keep an eye on the medicine cabinet. Also, make sure your child gets plenty of sleep, washes her hands and take other steps to stay generally healthy.

Despite all your best efforts, flares will seemingly appear out of nowhere. Among the steps that can help provide some relief:

- Apply an ice pack to your child's joints to help numb the joints and ease swelling. Apply cold in 20-minute sessions; then wait at least 10 minutes in between.

- Rubbing the sore joint gently might relieve pain and muscle stiffness. Ask your doctor for any recommendations regarding massage.

- Consider backing off of intense or vigorous sports or physical activities like dance. But don't go overboard. Movement helps retain range of motion in the joints. See if changing to new activities that stress joints less can keep your child moving with less pain or risk of injury. Be sure to let your child's doctor know.

- If the problem is joint contractures, splinting at night might help keep the joint correctly positioned during sleep. Be careful to use the splints as prescribed, because extensive immobilization of joints may cause stiffness.

- Make sure your child has a good sounding board for her flare-related fears and frustrations. Whether it's a close friend or a support group, she needs a safe outlet to share and talk with peers who know what she is going through.

"in remission" based on a doctor's physical exam, there may be ongoing disease that continues on a molecular level. (For this reason, your doctor may keep your child on medication long after she appears symptom-free.)

Plus, perception of remission may be relative. One study found that while doctors may diagnose inactive disease, only two-thirds of parents came to a similar conclusion, in part because the child still experienced pain or functional limitations. The researchers suggested that parental perceptions should be considered for inclusion in the recently designed remission criteria.

Assessing Likelihood of Remission for Your Child

What's the chance your child will go into remission? Since the JIA criteria on remission are relatively new, it's hard to determine the odds. One frequently cited analysis, from 2005 determined that 44 percent of the 437 patients studied experienced clinical remission off medication at least once.

The researchers, however, identified some significant differences by JIA type. Children with persistent oligoarticular JIA — those in which the arthritis remained in four or fewer joints — spent nearly 60 percent of the follow-up period in inactive disease. In several other groups of patients — those with systemic, extended oligoarthritis or rheumatoid factor (RF)-negative polyarthritis — the period of inactive disease was shorter, comprising 30 to 36 percent of the time studied. Children with polyarticular RF-positive disease were least likely; they experienced inactive disease 16 percent of the time.

Researchers also found that neither the age at diagnosis nor a positive test for ANA had any significant impact on an increased likelihood of remission off medication.

Meanwhile, sustained remission off medication proved elusive, according to the study's researchers. Once a child achieved clinical remission off medication, her chance of a flare within two years ranged from 40 to

GETTING RELIEF: TREATMENT GOALS
Your child's treatment goals, as well as how they are achieved, will require more than just pills or shots. When assessing whether her treatment is working, consider all aspects:

Goal: **Reduce inflammation.**
Strategies: Make sure she takes her prescribed medication faithfully.

Goal: **Ease pain.**
Strategies: Along with taking medication, try heat or cold treatments, relaxation techniques and exercise therapy.

Goal: **Stay flexible.**
Strategies: Use exercise to help prevent your child's stiffness and loss of motion.

Goal: **Get involved.**
Strategies: Make sure your child's illness doesn't prevent her from enjoying an active life — from school to hobbies to friends.

ENJOYING A REMISSION
Krystal Dudek's Story

Since Krystal Dudek was diagnosed with arthritis at 18 months, her life has been marked by periods of treatment separated by periods of remission, when the disease becomes inactive. The methotrexate and steroid injections can be set aside — for a time at least.

Telling when her disease is active or inactive, though, is far from easy. Krystal, an athletic 12-year-old, refuses to complain, as her mother, Carolyn, describes it. "She'll wake up in the morning limping and I'll say, 'Krystal—what is wrong?' And she'll say, 'Nothing.' I'll persist and ask again, 'What's wrong with your leg?' And she'll say: 'It's just really tired, Mom.'"

So several times a year, the family travels to Children's Hospital & Regional Medical Center in Seattle for checkups. And her mother tries to be optimistic, but not too hopeful, while their pediatric rheumatologist examines Krystal joint by joint. One time, when Krystal's parents thought their daughter was free of symptoms, her doctor pointed to a swollen toe on one foot. "We've hoped and we've had some disappointment," Carolyn says.

But the family also has enjoyed a healthy portion of good news, Carolyn is quick to say. By age 12, Krystal was enjoying her fourth remission, the previous three of which had persisted about a year and a half. Her current remission has stretched two years and counting, including 20 months off medication.

Krystal's only soreness involves her knees. But imaging tests indicate that the cause is probably athletic stresses, her mother says. (Krystal is constantly on the move, playing basketball, soccer and volleyball.)

Thankfully, Krystal's symptoms didn't reappear during the holidays, which had been a common pattern, says her mother.

So they nervously await each checkup, trying not to wish for too much. They know the odds remain long for a sustained remission—the pill bottles expiring in the medicine cabinet—but it *can* happen, they periodically remind themselves.

"I just got done asking her doctor a few weeks ago, 'Can I hope again?'" Carolyn recalls. "And she said: 'Yes, you can hope again.'"

> "Her current remission has stretched two years and counting, including 20 months off medication."

69 percent. Only 6 percent of medication-free remissions persisted more than five years. So it's likely your child will have to keep taking medications or at least restart them at some point.

Challenges and Hope Ahead

Still, it's important to remember that any remission analysis is merely a snapshot in time.

The 2005 study examined two decades prior to the routine usage of biologic medications. Ongoing studies are now scrutinizing the relative long-term benefit of not only individual biologic drugs, but also combinations of two or more classes of drugs.

Increasingly, pediatric rheumatologists say the challenge these days is less and less about achieving inactive disease. Rather, it's about maintaining that state of calm on the lowest doses of medication possible. One leading physician reports that she can achieve inactive disease in 80 percent of her patients with juvenile idiopathic arthritis by identifying the most effective combination of medications for that child. The difficulty, she says, is peeling away those medicines without the symptoms reappearing.

Not every child achieves the same level of relief, but don't give up hope. Work with your child's doctor to identify the combination of medications that minimizes your child's symptoms, if not completely eliminate them. And time is on your side. With every passing year, as researchers learn more, doctors may be able to pinpoint more successful treatments that lead to sustained remission off medication for increasing numbers of children with JIA. ●

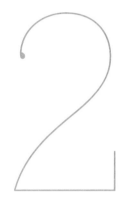

Medical Treatments and Strategies

Medication treatment in juvenile arthritis has changed dramatically in recent decades, both in terms of the drugs themselves and how they are prescribed. We'll explain why rheumatologists are striving to use medications earlier and more aggressively in the disease process. We'll provide a primer about the different classes of arthritis drugs, along with the surgical options available, if your child's disease progresses to that point. Other interventions will be detailed, including steps to help protect your child's eyes and jaw from arthritis-related damage.

....

CHAPTER SIX

Medications: Nuts and Bolts

For decades, treating juvenile arthritis (JA) with medications—and, in particular, treating what was then called juvenile rheumatoid arthritis—wasn't necessarily viewed with the same degree of urgency it is today. Some educational publications even carried the misleading claim that many children would simply grow out of this autoimmune disease. Thus, treatment was more likely to be approached in a stair-step fashion, with medications gradually added until symptom relief was achieved. We now know that this is not the best strategy, and you'll likely find that your physician will adopt a more aggressive stance to treating your child's arthritis.

How did we go from the wait-and-see approach of the past to the more targeted, assertive tactics of today?

In the early 1990s, a series of analyses and editorials began to turn the traditional treatment strategy for juvenile arthritis upside down. It became obvious that not treating the disease with agressively disease-modifying medications would lead to poor—and possibly permanent—outcomes. After a startling 1992 study, researchers found that as many as one-third to one-half of the kids they observed were still experiencing the effects of active disease 10 years or more after diagnosis. So doctors changed their approach. Increasingly, a diagnosis of juvenile rheumatoid arthritis (now called juvenile idiopathic arthritis) was recognized for the lifelong disabling threat that it poses, rather than an illness a child would outgrow with time.

By the mid-90s, physicians started recommending earlier and more aggressive treatment, including use of drugs once viewed as potentially toxic (such as methotrexate) in children who appeared the most vulnerable to joint damage. In this way, doctors hoped to intervene before permanent joint deformity and other serious outcomes developed.

In the years since, juvenile idiopathic arthritis (JIA) has been attacked on two fronts—with intervention earlier in the disease process and more sophisticated drugs. Where physicians once had to rely on aspirin, non-steroidal anti-inflammatory drugs (NSAIDs) and gold compounds, now they enjoy an ever-expanding array of drug options approved for adults first, and then used in children with arthritis. The late 1990s brought the new era of biologics, drugs that target the cells and related proteins of the immune system itself. In recent years, incentives for pharmaceutical companies also have fueled more testing of medications in children, providing better insights into dosages, side effects and other potential issues affecting this unique disease population.

The breakthroughs have been pronounced, in terms of better joint functioning and quality of life. With the more aggressive medication approach of today, children may take one individual drug or two or more in combination, and they experience substantially reduced symptoms and disabilities, both in the near term and down the road.

Today, parents and physicians have a clear goal of working to prevent even low-grade arthritis from smoldering unchecked. As a result, surgical replacement of joints, wrist-bone fusion and other procedures are far less common than they once were. For more children, remission is within grasp.

Still, you and your child's doctor will wrestle with the same thorny dilemma. How aggressively should your child's symptoms be treated, given the uncertain, long-term progression of the disease and the potential side effects of these new powerful drugs? Add to that mix other factors, including insurance coverage and the unique challenges of treating children, and designing your child's treatment plan can be difficult indeed.

Weighing Treatment Strategies

Every medication decision involves its own set of complex calculations, the balancing of relative risks and benefits that you must discuss with your child's doctor. The type of disease your child has may be influential. Children with polyarthritis who test positive for rheumatoid factor, for example, generally face a greater risk of long-term joint damage. Also, doctors may have differing treatment approaches, shaped by their practice style and your personal input.

Depending on the severity of your child's symptoms, some physicians may recommend initially, at least, the more traditional stair-step approach, beginning with a milder class of medication first, such as nonsteroidal anti-inflammatory drugs (NSAIDs), and then changing or adding to that regimen over time, until relief is achieved. With that approach, the physician has the advantage of knowing how your child reacts to each drug, both in terms of symptom relief and side effects. Insurance coverage also may play a role. Some policies require certain classes of drugs to be tried (and fail), before approving the use of more reliably effective but costly medications. The risk, though, is that your child's disease is worsening with time. Delaying the more aggressive drug treatment may, for some children, increase their risk of permanent joint damage or inflammation in vital organs.

That is why pediatric rheumatologists are increasingly adopting a step-down approach, moving aggressively from the moment of diagnosis. They hope to hit the arthritis early and hard, derailing the inflammatory cascade just as it begins to gain traction. Once the disease has been contained, the physician can pare back the medication until your child is taking the minimal amount necessary to maintain inactive disease.

This strategy is driven in part by intriguing results in adults with rheumatoid arthritis, which indicates that aggressive use of medications early in the course of the disease can result in less joint damage and a higher

....

A NEW PRESCRIPTION: SOME QUESTIONS TO ASK

Given the complexities and potential side effects involved with medication treatment, don't be hesitant to ask questions when your doctor suggests a new medication. Among some questions you could ask:

- Why are you prescribing this medication?

- How often should it be taken, and when?

- How long will it take to determine if the medication is working?

- Are there any special instructions, such as taking the medication with food?

- What are the possible side effects of this treatment?

- What should I do if I suspect a side effect?

- What steps should I take if my child misses a dose?

rate of remission than a more conservative course of treatment. Whether children with JIA can achieve similar results remains unclear.

In the meantime, if your physician cannot determine the optimal treatment path for your child's diagnosis, he or she may adopt a hybrid strategy. Your child may begin taking a milder class of drugs and then be quickly switched if they don't significantly reduce her symptoms. During this process, your input will be crucial. Don't hesitate to talk frankly with your child's doctor about your various fears and concerns. Ask yourself: How much do you fear drug side effect risks compared with the risks of your child's arthritis hurtling forward unchecked?

Over time, inflammation can irreversibly damage bone, cartilage and other tissues. Medication shouldn't be viewed as a guaranteed cure-all. Despite today's more effective drugs, some children with arthritis will remain frustratingly resistant to treatment. More often that not, though, you should notice substantial improvement in your child's symptoms—or better yet, complete control—within three to six months after diagnosis, as her physician strives to identify the best medication regimen. If your child hasn't enjoyed significant relief, raise your concerns to your doctor, or consider seeking a second opinion—even if it's long distance.

Pediatric Challenges and Risks

Treating kids with medications carries its own set of complex challenges, beginning with some of the psychological and lifestyle issues involved. As your child moves into adolescence, she may rebel outright, refusing to continue with her pills or weekly shots. Or her resistance may be more subtle, such as skipping doses. Your teen may become distracted by the increased social opportunities and pressures of high school and just get sloppy with her meds.

You also may contend with a new set of potential drug interactions. Despite your cautions otherwise, your teenager may experiment with alcohol, drugs or sexual activity without telling you or her doctor, while taking powerful medications for her JA. Teens with arthritis are still, at heart, teenagers, and they experience the same desires, temptations and social pressures that all teens face. And they don't like to confess everything that they are doing to their parents or doctors—just like other teens!

Then there are the risks of the medications themselves. One potential concern is that children's bodies are a work in progress and the immune system of very young children isn't fully developed. For that reason, some researchers worry that powerful immune-suppressing drugs like the biologics might have some effect on the immune system's maturation, although no data yet indicates this is a valid concern. Another worry involves the heightened risk of infection, given that children are exposed to plenty of germs. For that reason, your child's doctor may delay starting a biologic or advise skipping a dose if your child is battling an infection serious enough to require an antibiotic, antiviral or anti-fungal medication.

Medications A to Z: Class by Class

Listed below are some of the types of drugs your child may be taking now or down the road:

BIOLOGICS abatacept (*Orencia*), adalimumab (*Humira*), anakinra (*Kineret*), etanercept (*Enbrel*), infliximab (*Remicade*) and rituximab (*Rituxan*)

Considered the newest class in arthritis treatment, these biologic agents provide inflammatory relief by targeting some of the underpinnings of the immune system itself. Depending upon the drug involved, they either target specific cells—such as T cells or B cells—or proteins made by immune cells, such as tumor necrosis factor (TNF) or interleukin-1.

Adalimumab, etanercept and infliximab work by blocking TNF proteins, and the related messages to your immune system that help trigger inflammation. Anakinra blocks interleukin-1.

Abatacept and rituximab attempt to halt the inflammatory sequence earlier in the process by targeting cells that are activated before TNF or interleukin-1 proteins are made.

Biologics are costly and require either an injection or an intravenous infusion.

Side effects vary depending upon the drug, but can include reactions at the injection site, stomach problems, chills and fever. More seriously, by suppressing the immune system response, these drugs can increase risk of infection. For that reason, talk to your child's doctor before she receives any live vaccines. (*See sidebar, page 52.*)

At this time, there remains some uncertainty regarding biologics and long-term cancer risk. Because the drugs manipulate the immune system's regulation, the concern is that it may be less able to catch cancer cells at an

VACCINES: ISSUES TO CONSIDER

Vaccines, typically required for school or childcare admission, can involve a somewhat more complex set of decisions when your child has arthritis.

To date, the bulk of concern has involved live vaccines and how they interact with the child's immune system. The risks are by no means clear-cut, and a few recent studies indicate that some worries might be unfounded. It's preferable, however, to be cautious and review any vaccines carefully with your rheumatologist first.

Childhood immunizations are designed to work by essentially tricking the immune system, exposing your child to a very small dose of the relevant virus or bacteria. That trial run, so to speak, teaches your immune system how to combat the infection.

Arthritis or the medications your child is taking, such as methotrexate or the newer biologic agents, may already have altered her immune system to some degree. The vaccine may not work or your child could develop the disease itself. Or your child's arthritis could worsen.

Those vaccines referred to as live contain a live, but much weakened strain of the disease-causing organism. They include vaccines for chicken pox (varicella); measles, mumps and rubella (MMR); rotavirus and the nasal flu vaccine, *FluMist*. Many other vaccines contain strains of virus that have been killed, or inactivated. The polio vaccine contains an inactive form of the polio virus; so does the hepatitis A vaccine.

Worries about live vaccines may not be borne out. A 2007 study, looking at the use of the MMR vaccine in 314 children with juvenile idiopathic arthritis didn't identify any measles infection or notable increase in arthritis activity.

In light of the uncertainty, though, some pediatric rheumatologists prefer to err on the side of caution, not administering live vaccines in children currently taking immunosuppressive medications. Ideally, the vaccine delay is only temporary. The disease protection that immunization provides is even more beneficial for a child already battling a chronic illness like arthritis.

In the meantime, your child doesn't have to sit out of school. Your state will offer a medical exception for cases such as these, in which a doctor recommends against immunization.

To further protect your child, make sure other family members keep up with their shots. Take your child to the doctor immediately if she shows symptoms of illness. Antiviral medications are available for some diseases, including chickenpox and influenza. If begun within 48 hours of your child's symptoms, the antivirals hopefully will limit the severity of her illness.

early stage. The data from studies involving TNF blockers show a slightly higher, but still very rare, risk of lymphoma, a cancer of the immune system. Any cancer risk, if it does exist, may not be the same across all biologics because they don't all work in the same way.

CORTICOSTEROIDS methylprednisolone (*Medrol, Solumedrol*), prednisone (*Deltasone, Orapred, Orasone, Pediapred, Prelone, Sterapred*)

One of the older and faster-acting drugs used to treat arthritis and other inflammatory disease, corticosteroids (also called glucocorticoids or cortisone-like drugs) are typically used with special care in children. Corticosteroids are hormones naturally produced by the adrenal gland—a gland located above the kidney—that help suppress inflammation and the immune system. Synthetic forms, such as prednisone tablets or prednisolone syrups can be prescribed for oral administration to combat systemic inflammation. Injections can be delivered directly into a joint to reduce local inflammation. A common form of eye inflammation, called uveitis, is treated with steroid eye drops.

If prescribed for systemic use, the lowest dosage of corticosteroid will typically be given for the shortest period possible to minimize common side effects, such as weight gain and mood swings. To limit the dose, your child's doctor also may prescribe another drug, such as methotrexate.

Other potential side effects with long-term usage of corticosteroids include easier bruising, a moon-shaped face, acne, osteoporosis, facial hair growth and cataracts. Because higher doses of corticosteroids can suppress your immune system, the medications also can sometimes increase your child's vulnerability to infections.

Corticosteroids should be taken exactly as prescribed. It should not be stopped nor the dosage decreased without a doctor's direction; in fact, it may be dangerous to stop a corticosteroid suddenly. To minimize side effects of long-term use of corticosteroids, it's very important that your child eats a healthy diet and exercises. Calcium and vitamin D supplements also may be recommended.

To treat an individual joint or a couple of joints, the doctor injects a corticosteroid compound, sometimes along with an anesthetic for immediate pain relief, directly into the inflamed joint. If the joint has a lot of fluid in it, the doctor might drain the fluid from the joint before injecting the

TWO MEDICATION MIRACLES
Bridget Boockmeier's Story

Andy Boockmeier and his wife, Annie, have witnessed the power of medication—twice—since their daughter, Bridget, was diagnosed with polyarthritis shortly before her fourth birthday.

First she was started on an NSAID, but that didn't seem to make a significant dent in her pain and inflammation. On her worst days, the Chicago girl struggled to rise from bed, her legs shaking once they hit the ground. Her parents would carry her downstairs.

So Bridget's physician started the little girl on methotrexate, warning that a month or more might pass before it took effect. But in just a few weeks, the payoff was clear. Andy vividly recalls the morning when Bridget got out of bed and began kicking her legs into the air "like a drum major."

Fast forward two years; Bridget had hit another painful wall. "It got her everywhere a joint possibly could," says Andy, recounting that August stretch. By September, Bridget's physician had administered the first shot of etanercept (*Enbrel*). Again, they were cautioned not to expect too much too fast.

"The next morning she got up, put on her gym clothes and bounded down the stairs for breakfast and got onto her chair without a bit of help," Andy says.

"I remember asking her, 'Do your knees hurt?,'" he recalls. "And she said, 'No.' And I said, 'Do your fingers hurt?' And she said, 'No.' And I said, 'How does your neck feel?' She turns it from side to side and says: 'It feels fine.'"

"My wife and I, we couldn't even say anything. Our eyes were full of tears."

Andy sometimes gets asked about the powerful drugs his daughter takes and whether he worries about the uncertainties associated with their long-term effects.

"You have to put that stuff behind you," he says. "Right now the most important thing is getting my daughter's health under control and I feel like we're there. I pray that this [medication regimen] won't have a long-term effect on her. But right now her body and her joints and just her overall well-being need this medicine just to feel healthy."

Her parents have become astute at catching the subtle signs of a developing flare. She tends to sleep a lot more. She's less interested in eating, more likely to turn down a snack. She'll start asking for piggy back rides. But rarely does she complain.

"She is 7 years old and has dealt with adult-sized pain for three years," Andy says. "I refer to her as a warrior because of what she has endured."

medication. Injections can be done in any joint, but are most commonly delivered to the knee. There's virtually no recovery time involved.

If the injection successfully reduces inflammation, the need for other medications is diminished. Not all steroid preparations are equivalent, so be sure you are getting one well-recognized for its effectiveness for arthritis in children. Frequent injections may not be optimal therapy. Some doctors may recommend you consider other options if your child needs the same joints injected multiple times annually.

DISEASE-MODIFYING ANTIRHEUMATIC DRUGS (DMARDs) azathioprine (*Imuran*), cyclosporine (*Neoral*), hydroxychloroquine sulfate (*Plaquenil*), leflunomide (*Arava*), methotrexate (*Rheumatrex, Trexall*), sulfasalazine (*Azulfidine*)

These drugs do not produce an immediate relief in pain or inflammation, but are believed (hence the class name) to modify the natural course of the disease and prevent joint damage. Depending upon the drug, they can take anywhere from one to three months, and possibly longer, to show results. Since the benefits of a DMARD might not kick in for a couple of months, your child's doctor might also prescribe another drug, such as a corticosteroid or an NSAID, to provide faster inflammatory relief. Only a few of the drugs, including leflunomide (*Arava*) and sulfasalazine (*Azulfidine*) were developed specifically to treat rheumatoid arthritis. Others first showed their benefits in other areas of medicine. (*See sidebar, page 56.*) Hydroxychloroquine is a malaria drug, for example, and methotrexate was initially a chemotherapy treatment.

At least two-thirds of children with persistently active juvenile idiopathic arthritis require some type of DMARD, according to a review of JIA treatment published 2006. Methotrexate has become an increasingly common weapon of choice, used earlier and more effectively. It provides a beneficial effect about 70 percent of the time.

Side effects can vary among DMARDs—some detail is provided below—but they all have the potential to suppress your child's immune system to some degree. That's why it's important to alert your child's doctor if she develops an infection. Also, check before getting any live vaccines, such as the MMR or varicella (chickenpox) vaccines. As with most medications, it also is important for children of child-bearing age to discuss pregnancy risks and birth control with their doctor, who can explain the effect of certain medications on a fetus.

Some examples of other side effects, depending upon the DMARD, include:

Azathioprine (*Imuran*): Given in pill form, this should be taken with food. Side effects may include fever or chills, loss of appetite, nausea and liver problems.

MEDICATIONS: BORROWING FROM OTHER ILLNESSES

Many of the drugs your child routinely takes to treat her juvenile arthritis weren't even developed specifically for the autoimmune disease.

Methotrexate, now considered a staple treatment in juvenile arthritis, was originally conceived and continues to be used as a cancer chemotherapy treatment, albeit in dramatically higher dosages. Cyclosporine (*Neoral*) was originally prescribed to prevent transplant recipients from rejecting their newly acquired organs. More recently, mycophenolate mofetil (*CellCept*), another antirejection drug, has become a crucial tool in combating lupus. The list of so-called borrowed drugs could stretch on and on.

So parents face a difficult dilemma. The typical advice is for consumers to be cautious about the use of "off-label" drugs. A medication is considered off label if it's being prescribed for a condition other than the one for which it was specifically tested. Once approved, though, doctors are free to prescribe it off-label for other diseases or age groups, based on data and clinical experience indicating that it could be helpful.

In serious diagnoses, such as juvenile arthritis, off-label treatments have traditionally been the norm rather than the exception. That's partly because doctors were striving to identify better treatments to short-circuit inflammation and its consequences. Drug testing in children historically has been very limited. Until the federal government and Congress started implementing requirements and incentives for such testing, pharmaceutical companies had little incentive to conduct the research.

The consequence: Some of the ground-breaking advances in arthritis treatment have been derived from other classes of drugs. Borrowing from existing drugs for treatment of juvenile arthritis persists, particularly in cases where other treatments haven't given significant relief and your child's doctor remains concerned about long-term joint damage. So when should you consider expanding treatment beyond the typical regimens?

Cyclosporine (*Neoral*): Side effects may include headache, increased hair growth, loss of appetite, nausea and kidney problems. Because the drug's absorption is sometimes variable, your child might need periodic blood tests to monitor levels. Avoid St. John's wort, grapefruit or grapefruit juice.

Hydroxychloroquine sulfate (*Plaquenil*): This drug is given in pill form and should be taken with food to avoid stomach upset. Side effects may include upset stomach, headache or rash. High doses used for diseases other

If your child's doctor suggests borrowing from another class, don't hesitate to clarify exactly why. You might want to ask how often that drug has been used in children with juvenile arthritis, as well as how often the doctor has used that particular drug. Are you still unsure? You can always request a second opinion. As with any medication, once your child starts taking the new drug, make sure you're well-briefed on dosage issues and potential side effects so you can watch for any early signs of trouble.

Borrowing in juvenile arthritis occurs across a number of drug classes, but here are two recent examples your doctor might suggest or that you may hear about in discussions with other parents:

ACNE DRUGS: Acne drugs in the tetracycline family have been used in adults with rheumatoid arthritis. As a result, the drugs—primarily minocycline (*Minocin*)—have been prescribed to some children with the childhood equivalent of adult RA (rheumatoid factor-positive polyarthritis). The drug is believed to work by decreasing the production of substances, such as metalloproteinases, that cause inflammation. Children must be closely monitored for side effects, which can include stomach problems, a rash and, more rarely, illnesses that resemble lupus.

SLEEP AIDS: Thalidomide, a sedative drug, gained notoriety when it caused birth defects in the 1950s and 1960s after doctors prescribed it to prevent morning sickness and sleeping problems in pregnant women. Researchers have continued to work with the drug and, in recent years, it's been approved for limited use to treat a couple of conditions, including leprosy and multiple myeloma. Thalidomide also is being used in systemic JIA, typically after other treatments have failed. The sedative drug is believed to have some similar mechanisms to biologic drugs, working in part by blocking TNF. Other molecules are believed to be blocked as well, including interleukin-6. Side effects can include constipation and sleepiness. Because of its birth defects history, the drug's use is tightly regulated.

BEATING INFLAMMATION
Julie Smith's Essay

Gavin was 22 months old when he was diagnosed with juvenile arthritis. It started with a swollen knee the month before and his doctor told us to see an orthopedic surgeon. That day we went, they took X-rays and said they think he fractured his growth plate. They put on a cast for four weeks.

After four weeks, when they took the cast off his knee, it was three times its original size and he was screaming in pain. They drained some fluid and for the first time, it was arthritis. Then they sent us to a pediatric rheumatologist at All Children's Hospital in Tampa.

Gavin was put on naproxen that day. His knee was so swollen and in so much pain that he kept it at a 90 degree angle and stopped walking.

At his second visit, the pediatric rheumatologist suggested steroid injections. By then, his wrist also was swollen and he wasn't using it. So Gavin received injections in both joints.

Two weeks later, the doctor wasn't happy with the results. My son was still not walking and his wrist was even worse.

The doctor started Gavin on methotrexate injections once a week. He told us it would take at least a month before we would see any results.

That night I gave him his first injection, and the next day my son started taking tiny steps! The day after that, he walked more than he crawled! It has been only three days since the methotrexate injection and he's doing awesome.

He walks with a limp and not for very long, but he is walking! Soon, he will start physical therapy to build up the muscles in his leg again.

> "I can't tell you how good it feels to see that smile on his face when he stands up on his own and walks."

I can't tell you how good it feels to see that smile on his face when he stands up on his own and walks.

I just wanted to tell my story in case someone is feeling like there is no light at the end of the tunnel like I did. Just so you know: There is light at the end of the tunnel and it is the most beautiful light I have ever seen.

—*Julie Smith, lives in Tampa, Fla. Her son, Gavin, is 2 years old.*

than arthritis have been associated with effects on the eyes, but doses for rheumatic diseases have been demonstrated to be safe. A special yearly eye exam will be recommended to be certain it is used safely.

Methotrexate (*Rheumatrex*): This drug is taken weekly either by pill or injection. Side effects may include decreased appetite, nausea, mouth sores, mild hair thinning, fatigue, lung irritation (cough), increased sun sensitivity and liver problems. Methotrexate can deplete levels of the vitamin folic acid, and this can increase the likelihood of these side effects occurring, so folic acid supplementation (such as a multivitamin or folic acid tablets) may be recommended. Your doctor will also recommend avoiding other irritants for the lungs (smoking) or liver (alcohol). Your child's doctor will order liver tests and blood cell counts before starting the drug and then repeat the tests to monitor for any side effects. Contraception is often required for people of child-bearing age taking this medication.

Sulfasalazine (*Azuldifine*): This medication is given in pill form, typically twice a day. Side effects may include stomach upset, headache, increased sun sensitivity and low white blood cell counts.

NONSTEROIDAL ANTI-INFLAMMATORY DRUGS (NSAIDs) Among other effects, NSAIDs block the production of prostaglandins, which are hormone-like substances that contribute to pain, inflammation, fever and muscle cramps. When used in low doses, NSAIDs can ease aches and fever. In larger doses, the medications can reduce redness and swelling in your child's joints. They can be prescribed in many different forms: pills, suppositories, liquids and injections.

NSAIDs are typically broken down into two classes: traditional NSAIDs and a newer class, called selective COX-2 inhibitors.

TRADITIONAL NSAIDs: aspirin (*Anacin, Bayer, Bufferin, Exedrin*, etc.), choline magnesium salicylate (*Trilisate*), diclofenac sodium (*Voltaren*), ibuprofen (*Advil, Motrin*), indomethacin (*Indocin*), meloxicam (*Mobic*), nabumetone (*Relafen*), naproxen (*Naprosyn*), piroxicam (*Feldene*), salsalate (*Disalcid*) and sulindac (*Clinoril*), among others

In cases of mild arthritis, taking an NSAID may be sufficient for relief of pain and inflammation. NSAIDs typically come in pill or liquid form, and are taken one to four times daily. Your child may take the medication for at least a month before it helps limit her discomfort.

HERBAL SUPPLEMENTS: DECISIONS AND OPTIONS

Perhaps your sister passed along an interesting article. Or an advertisement caught your eye, touting an "all-natural" remedy for arthritis symptoms. Within a few days, you're roaming the shelves of a nearby pharmacy or natural-foods store searching for the silver bullet to end your child's inflammatory miseries. When your child is dealing with pain, inflammation, and other devastating symptoms of juvenile arthritis, you will do anything to bring her relief. But when it comes to complementary therapies, it's very important to proceed carefully and keep your doctor informed.

An estimated one-third of children with JIA have used a complementary or alternative treatment at some point, ranging from acupuncture to dietary supplements to massage, according to a recent study. Despite the attractive labels, though, the decision to start your child on fish oils, glucosamine or another type of herbal supplement should be reached carefully and in consultation with your child's arthritis specialist.

For all herbal supplements, there are some basic cautions to keep in mind. Since the products aren't federally regulated like prescription medications are, there's no guarantee that what's described on the outside of the bottle—such as the dosage of the key ingredient—is inside the packaging. Also, use caution when assessing the stated health claims. Do your own digging to find out what researchers have learned about the nutrient or herb involved. And don't be falsely soothed by the assertion that the key ingredients are "natural." Some powerful prescribed medications are derived from plants, such as the heart drug digitalis, which comes from the foxglove plant.

Herbal supplements are frequently described as complementary treatment because it's assumed they are being added to your child's prescribed medication regimen. But your child shouldn't start swallowing any new pills, however innocuous they may seem, without talking first to her physician.

Even if the doctor is comfortable with adding the supplement, your child's other medication may need to be adjusted as a result. So it's important to be upfront about your interest; don't postpone having that conversation. In other cases, the proposed herbal supplement could undercut some of the benefits of your child's existing medications. For example, some medications—echinacea is one—are typically taken to boost the body's immune system. But in people with arthritis, the treatment goal is more to blunt the edge of an over-active immune system.

Herbal supplement use in children raises yet another set of unknowns, given the ongoing development of their young bodies. Most research involves adults, not kids. Take glucosamine and chondroitin sulfate, two substances that are widely marketed to help rebuild cartilage, for example. Although they are safe in adults, some concerns have been raised by doctors about children taking the substances and incorporating them into their bones while they are still growing.

If you want to investigate a particular treatment, the National Center for Complementary and Alternative Medicine posts recent studies, along with a detailed health glossary, at **http://nccam.nih.gov.** In 2005, the institute published a research report that's available online: "Rheumatoid Arthritis and Complementary and Alternative Medicine." The Arthritis Foundation also published a comprehensive A-to-Z guide, *Alternative Treatments for Arthritis.*

In the meantime, listed below are several of the herbal supplements that you might see promoted for use in arthritis:

FISH OILS: There is some encouraging research on these oils, in terms of easing sore joints and morning stiffness. The extent of the effect, as well as which types of patients would benefit most, isn't fully known. Fish oils contain high amounts of two omega-3 fatty acids, EPA (eicosapentaneoic acid) and DHA (docosahexaenoic acid). Some fish species, including shark and swordfish, contain high levels of mercury, particularly worrisome in pregnant women and young children. So look for a product comprised from fish with low mercury levels (Check out the Seafood Water Program at Monterey Bay Aquarium, **www.monterybayaquarium.org**). Other side effects can include a fishy aftertaste and some stomach disturbances.

GAMMA-LINOLENIC ACID (GLA): **This** omega-6 fatty acid is found in some plant seeds, including evening primrose, borage and black currant. A review of seven studies found some association with improvement of joint tenderness and morning stiffness when compared to placebo-treated patients, although there were still some uncertainties. Taking supplements with GLA does carry some risks of interactions with other drugs. One possible risk is increased bleeding, if borage or evening primrose is mixed with blood-thinning drugs, including aspirin or nonsteroidal anti-inflammatory drugs (NSAIDs). Side effects can include diarrhea, gas and stomach bloating.

GLUCOSAMINE AND CHONDROITIN SULFATE: These substances, sold individually or in combination, are found in the fluid and cartilage in the joints. A National Institutes of Health study, involving nearly 1,600 participants with osteoarthritis in the knee, found that the combination did not provide significant relief overall. But those complaining of moderate to severe pain did report a meaningful difference. Side effects of the drugs include stomach problems and nausea. There is some concern that glucosamine could possibly decrease the effectiveness of certain medications, including acetaminophen, which is widely used in children for treating pain.

Although NSAIDs are a common sight in drug and grocery stores, with lower doses available over-the-counter, they do carry the potential for side effects. One of the biggest concerns is stomach problems, more likely if the NSAID is taken in large doses or for a long period of time. Some symptoms may include heartburn, stomach pain or nausea.

More importantly, NSAID use can increase the risk of developing a stomach ulcer. Some of the risk factors aren't as relevant to children. In particular, ulcers are more common in those over age 60, or with a chronic diseases of the heart, liver or kidneys. Drinking alcohol or smoking tobacco also elevates the risk of side effects, so it is very important for you to discuss the increased danger of experimenting with tobacco, alcohol or recreational drugs with your child if she takes these medications.

Your child's doctor may suggest several steps to protect her stomach, such as taking the NSAID with food or prescribing another medication (antacid or proton pump inhibitor) to soothe any stomach-related effects. It's also important for your child to get regular checkups and call a doctor if signs of a bleeding ulcer develop: bloody vomit, or black, tarry or bloody bowel movements.

Aspirin is rarely, if ever, used in children because there are other safer and more effective options. Not only is it associated with a dangerous complication called Reyes syndrome, but it also is believed to pose a greater risk than other NSAIDs for causing stomach upset and ulcers. Other types of related drugs, called non-acetylated or non-aspirin salicylates, are believed to cause less stomach upset and come with a lower risk of gastrointestinal bleeding.

COX-2 INHIBITORS: celecoxib (*Celebrex*)

This class of drugs was originally designed to provide the anti-inflammatory benefits of NSAIDs without as many associated risks to the stomach. In recent years, however, two of the three drugs in the class—rofecoxib (*Vioxx*) and valdecoxib (*Bextra*)—were withdrawn by manufacturers after concerns were raised based on research in adults. Celecoxib (*Celebrex*) has continued to be available for adults, and more recently was approved specifically for use in children, after careful review of newer research.

Vioxx received the most publicity after research showed an elevated risk of heart problems in adults, including heart attack and stroke. The drug's manufacturer voluntarily withdrew the drug in 2004. Shortly afterward, in

2005, Food and Drug Administration officials asked *Bextra*'s manufacturer to withdraw that drug based on similar cardiovascular reasons, as well as concerns about a potentially serious skin reaction. Federal officials also requested the addition of a black box warning to all prescription NSAID products, including *Celebrex*, citing the heart risks.

Research further assessing the relative risks and benefits of *Celebrex* is ongoing. Be sure to ask your child's doctor about the latest findings as they relate to the drug's relative risks and benefits in children.

Moving Forward

Historically, information about medication side effects, dosing issues and other concerns in children has been limited for two chief reasons. Until recently it has been difficult for medical centers to pool enough children with juvenile arthritis to sufficiently study the effects of various drug treatments. Plus, pharmaceutical companies didn't have a financial incentive to study drugs in children; virtually all of their research was confined to adults.

Since the late 1990s, those research constraints have been relaxed by a combination of legislation and research initiatives. In 1998, the Food and Drug Administration issued the Pediatric Rule, requiring pharmaceutical companies to test a new drug in children if the disease involved also

....

THE FDA PROCESS: GETTING APPROVAL

Years can pass before a new drug is approved by the U.S. Food and Drug Administration, with numerous benchmarks along the way. Once federally approved, your child's doctor can prescribe the drug for its stated purpose; insurance companies also are more likely to cover it. The drug also might be prescribed for other conditions when there's evidence of clinical benefit, typically referred to as off-label use.

What types of studies are required? Three phases of clinical trials are conducted. The earliest and generally smallest studies, called Phase I, focus on the drug's safety, side effects and how it's metabolized in the body. Phase II can't begin if there's indication of unacceptable toxicity. If research continues, Phase II collects some of the first information about the drug's effectiveness. The final phase, Phase III, is typically the largest study, with several hundred to three thousand participants. In this phase, the most detailed information is collected about safety, effectiveness and the relative benefit of the drug in different doses and different populations.

How are the studies designed? The clinical trials must be reviewed by FDA officials and a local institutional review board. Besides scrutinizing the study design itself, the institutional review board makes sure that individuals participating are fully informed of the risks and other protective steps are taken.

occurred in children. Although that rule was overturned by a federal judge several years later, it helped to kick start pediatric testing, assisting children with arthritis in the process.

In 2002, Congress passed the Best Pharmaceuticals for Children Act (BPCA), which gave pharmaceutical companies an incentive to test drugs in children by providing them an additional six months of patent exclusivity, prior to the approval of any generic alternatives. Patent exclusivity provides a company with exclusive rights to market and sell a particular drug before it can be manufactured generically and sold by many companies at cheaper prices. The act, which was renewed five years later, boosted the degree of attention pharmaceutical companies devoted to the drug's possible pediatric uses during the patenting process. From 2002 through 2005, pharmaceutical companies agreed to study 173 of the 214 on-patent drugs (81 percent) for which FDA officials submitted written requests, according to a 2007 Government Accountability Office report.

At the same time, researchers have been merging forces, forming national and international multicenter networks to more effectively conduct research on medication treatments and other issues. These groups include the Childhood Arthritis and Rheumatology Research Alliance, the Pediatric Rheumatology Collaborative Study Group and the Pediatric Rheumatology International Trials Organization, among others. The data and insights collected by such organizations hopefully will shed more light in the years ahead on the pluses and minuses of various medication classes.

As your child gets older, gains weight or develops side effects, her prescribed regimen will probably be tweaked or possibly even overhauled. Stay vigilant. You'll need the latest research data when you revisit your child's treatment options in the years ahead. Don't settle for your child enduring limited symptoms if you can squelch them entirely; be aggressive with your treatment approach. ●

....

CHAPTER SEVEN

Medication-Related Issues

Selecting a medication regimen for your child may seem like small potatoes compared with the ongoing challenges—week after week—of motivating her to take the joint-protecting drugs. To treat her arthritis, your child may be prescribed multiple medications, which may literally require a spread sheet to keep straight. Some of those drugs can involve injections, which have their own set of stressors.

Adhering to that medication schedule as you juggle work and other family responsibilities can be daunting. Besides the logistics, there also will be emotional challenges involved, whether it's coping with your small child's stubborn streak or the open revolt of a teenager grown weary of battling a chronic disease.

In the years ahead, you will adopt a variety of roles: cheerleader, support system, drug researcher and, yes, disciplinarian. You will learn how to handle aspects of parenthood that you never anticipated, such as giving injections. You will learn how to make tough calls, such as enrolling your child in a research trial. And you will learn how to let go, bit by bit. As your child gets older—and sooner than you might expect—she can start handling some aspects of her complex medication regimen. But you can never let down your guard. The stakes are too high.

Understanding the Basics

When it comes to getting the most out of your child's medication plan, consistency is key, but easier said than done. To be achieved, your child must understand not only why she's taking the medication, but why it's so crucial that she doesn't skip a dose. Explain in age-appropriate language what the medication is supposed to do. For a young child, you may simply state that the pills or shots will help her feel better. As your child gets older, you can be more specific about short-term benefits—better mobility on the soccer field—along with the longer-term protection for her joints that she may not fully appreciate at a young, short-sighted age.

To help your child stay on track, you can implement several strategies, beginning with setting a routine. Pick a specific time each day or each week to take the medication, keeping the rhythms of your child's schedule in mind. If she's old enough, sit down and discuss what time would best mesh with her home and school routine. A digital watch or programmed cell phone alarm could help out, beeping a reminder. Your child could reset it once she's taken her medication. Some parents will post a medication form prominently on the bathroom mirror or the refrigerator door. Once your child takes her pills or shot, she can apply a sticker or check off the appropriate box.

If she's keeping up, reward her with positive feedback. That may be as simple as praise—even sullen teenagers appreciate kudos—or more tangible rewards. You could develop a system in which your child compiles stickers or points of some kind. Once they accumulate, she can redeem them for a special activity, prize or a weekly allowance. Be creative and don't feel guilty that you're engaging in bribery. Yes, your child is supposed to take her medication, but she may not be sufficiently mature to understand the long-term risks of not taking it. A little positive reinforcement now is a small price to pay for better health later. Some children with arthritis may, at times, be unable to participate in the same sports, games or activities as their friends, so creating contests or goals for them, with successes celebrated, can really encourage them to stay on track.

Defusing Medication Fights

Rebellion can percolate in a variety of forms. Whining and complaining about taking medications can certainly become wearing, particularly over

PERSONAL STORY
....

STICKING WITH THE MEDS
Jessie Meng's Story

Jessie Meng only has vague memories of her years battling the systemic form of juvenile arthritis. But her parents won't ever forget those painful, seemingly endless, days.

Jessie, diagnosed near her first birthday, was so ill that she scarcely grew between her first and second birthdays, recalls her father, Michael Meng. For a couple of years, she sometimes needed to be carried because she found it too painful to walk. And Jessie visited the doctor constantly, sometimes every week, as her pediatric rheumatologist strived to find the right combination of medication.

What Jessie's physician recalls is how much her parents hated administering the drugs and, in particular, the injections—sometimes two or three a week. Michael would blanch when a new drug regimen was suggested. But he always squared his shoulders, saying he would do anything to help his daughter.

Still, some days were very discouraging. "During that time, I could almost not see the hope," Michael says.

Then Jessie reached age 2½ and her parents started getting small doses of good news.

Her blood work showed signs that the drugs were beating back the autoimmune disease. But her parents didn't see any changes in Jessie and then, at least initially, only slowly. By age 3, she didn't need to be carried any longer.

Then one morning, when Jessie was 3½, a magical day dawned.

"She stood up and started walking," her father recalls. "And then she started running—we could not believe it. She was running through the whole house."

Jessie's parents had never seen their little girl run before.

As the years passed, Jessie's doctor continued to very slowly reduce the number of drugs Jessie was taking, along with the dosages. The Minneapolis girl came in for checkups, but less frequently.

When Jessie was 9 years old, the doctor told her family that they didn't need to return, as long as she felt well. There are never any guarantees; Jessie's symptoms could reappear. For now, she's in extended remission off medication, her fevers and painful inflammation a fading memory.

Systemic arthritis can be a difficult disease to battle, particularly if the initial symptoms are severe. But the ending can sometimes be better than expected with the right medication and vigilant adherence to the prescribed treatment plan.

time. Try to ignore your child's protests as much as possible; don't lose your cool. Avoid getting drawn into an extended discussion, which can spill over into a full-out battle, leaving everyone drained and the medication sitting untouched on the bathroom counter.

Hopefully, the complaints will recede over time. When the griping gets tough, here are some strategies and wording you can employ:

- Use a sympathetic, but firm, approach. If your child complains, say: "I know you don't like taking your medication, but it's helping you."
- If your child persists, try to ignore her complaints as long as she eventually does take the medication.
- If you detect a change in attitude, such as less grumbling before taking the meds, reward that with praise.
- In the case of an older child, tell her that you don't want to argue and walk away. Thus you provide your child an opportunity to comply on her own.

Needless to say, you may encounter a day when you hit a brick wall. If your child refuses to cooperate, some form of discipline is your only option. While this may be particularly difficult, given that your child is already battling a chronic disease, it's important that you treat her like you would any stubborn or uncooperative child.

To best capture your child's attention, avoid emotional responses, such as pleading or yelling or spanking. Instead, set clear-cut rules and then follow through with consequences if they're not followed. And those consequences should be age-specific.

Younger children will respond well to some form of "time out." Have your child to sit in a boring place (no TV or computer) for a prescribed period of time; the younger the child, the shorter the requisite time. Once the timeout is over, ask her again to follow through with taking her medication. An older child may respond better to the withholding of a beloved privilege, such as computer or cell phone use for a day. After taking the medications the following day, she can earn those privileges back.

One potential hurdle to medication success: side effects. Pay attention to any complaints, particularly when your child starts a new medication. Some side effects can be minimized or eliminated. Your child's doctor could prescribe medication, for example, to ease stomach upset. If an injection is involved, it's particularly important to address side effects—if possible—early on. Otherwise your child may develop the side effect, such as nausea, as soon as she catches sight of the needle.

Giving Injections

Some medications are easier to take than others. When injections are involved, parents and children alike can approach the weekly ritual with equal dread. Let's face it: Nobody likes shots!

To reduce the anxiety of everyone involved, try to provide your child with a sense of control, where feasible. Allow her to select the time of day when the shot is given. Some children may develop their own personalized rituals, such as wearing a favorite hat or pair of shoes. One clinician described a girl who asked her parents to photograph various stages of the injection process. This allowed her to line the photos up ahead of time to visualize the process before administering her own shot.

Distraction also can be your child's friend. Younger children may want to blow bubbles. An older child may fare better while chatting with a close friend by phone. Again, try to offer opportunities for choice and control. If your child prefers to watch a television program or video, let her pick the show.

As you fine tune your approach, take queues from your child's body language to see how she's reacting. Some children may prefer to apply a skin-numbing cream to the area. But because the cream can take some time to work—as long as an hour—that delay may amplify your child's nerves. Similarly, while some children may want to see the shot prepared; others may want you to do it in another room.

If your child is fearful of the needle, a device called an auto-injector can hide the sharp point. In cases where your child's fear is extreme, you may need to take additional steps to slowly desensitize her. Start by asking her only to sit in the same room with the syringe. Later, you can ask her to hold it. Eventually, you'll add the needle. As your child becomes more accustomed to the equipment, her fear hopefully will recede.

What if you're struggling with your own injection-related fears? Pediatric rheumatology clinics typically offer training for parents, including videos and opportunities to practice. You may be able to convince a friend or family member with a medical background to step in until you're ready to take the responsibility. Possibly, a nearby medical clinic will give the weekly shot, for a fee. Whenever possible, try to shield your child from your anxiety because it will only amplify her own.

As time passes—and more quickly than you may realize—your child may be ready to handle giving herself her own shots. Doctors report that

---

PERSONAL ESSAY

LEARNING TO GIVE A SHOT
Tracy Freeman's Essay

Most people say, "Thank God It's Friday!" I say, "Ugh, It's Friday." Since our 4-year-old daughter, Cassidy, was diagnosed several months ago, Fridays have meant one thing: injection day.

While I do believe that Cassidy is getting world-class care, I was still dumbstruck when her doctor informed me that I would be responsible for administering her weekly methotrexate injection. They gave me a demonstration and an instructional DVD, and then I was on my own. Don't these people realize that I am not medically inclined? I couldn't even dissect a frog in high school!

For the first month I either took her to the pediatrician's office or recruited one of my nurse friends to give her the injection. Unfortunately, this just seemed to add to the trauma of the event. I knew that I would have to take our rheumatologist's advice and give Cassidy her injection at nighttime myself.

The first time I was a wreck. I couldn't even figure out how to take the cap off of the needle—that wasn't on the video! I practiced several times until I felt comfortable with it. My heart was beating so fast and my palms were sweaty. I put the *Emla* cream on her while she slept and hoped she would stay asleep during the shot, too.

However, as soon as the needle touched her arm, she jumped out of bed with limbs flailing. So my husband carried her to the living room and I gave her the injection. It was at least two hours before I could fall asleep after that.

Since then, it's gotten easier. But it's not easy. On the instructional DVD, the mother and daughter demonstrating the shot look so happy and relaxed. We're not there yet, but I'm confident that we will be.

— Tracy Freeman and Cassidy,
who has juvenile psoriatic arthritis,
live in Ponca City, Okla.

---

children as young as first- or second-graders have developed the requisite control and other skills to be able to give themselves shots. Self-administering the injection may provide your child a newfound sense of control, both literal and psychological. On her own, your child can make subtle, instinctual adjustments as she delivers the medication, preventing the process from being painful. At the same time, she has taken a very significant step forward in tackling the medical management of her own disease. In fact, she may never want someone else to touch the needle again.

Considering a Clinical Trial

When no medication regimen controls your child's symptoms, you may be offered another route: the opportunity to participate in a clinical research trial. Many of today's best treatments first emerged from, or were validated by, research studies. Even so, you will have a lot of questions before deciding whether this is the best decision for your family.

At any given time, numerous research trials are available, with varying types of focus and design. Some trials look at ways to prevent diseases whereas others weigh the relative effectiveness of screening and diagnostic tools. Medication studies are considered treatment trials and they scrutinize individual drugs or combinations of drugs. Most, if not all, medications approved for adults with rheumatoid arthritis are being studied in children.

In some respects, a research trial can offer practical advantages. Besides gaining access to cutting-edge medication and its potential benefit, your child will be contributing to important research insights. Participants in clinical research trials also are closely followed. Your child will receive comprehensive medical care during the course of the trial and some, if not all, of the costs will likely be covered.

At the same time, don't ignore the potential drawbacks. There's no guarantee that the medication will work and there's always the risk of side effects. The monitoring involved may require an additional time commitment for clinic visits and extra laboratory screening, such as blood tests.

If the study involves a placebo medication, your child will be randomly assigned to take the medication under scrutiny or the placebo (sugar pill). Some studies are described as blinded, which means that you won't know what medication your child is receiving. Even if your child is getting an injection, it could be of saline or another placebo substance—tinted or

PERSONAL STORY

TRYING THE TREAT TRIAL
Daina Faust's Story

Daina Faust's parents left the decision in her hands.

The 9-year-old girl, who lives near Seattle, had just been diagnosed with polyarthritis. Her pediatric rheumatologist provided an option. Did she want to participate in a clinical trial, designed to test an aggressive medication intervention?

Dubbed TREAT, the trial is called Trial of Early Aggressive Drug Therapy in Juvenile Idiopathic Arthritis. It's considered one of the best ongoing research efforts to determine whether hitting the autoimmune disease with an aggressive regimen shortly after diagnosis can trigger clinical remission. That approach has shown some success in adults with rheumatoid arthritis, but findings aren't yet available in children.

For Daina, it didn't take much second guessing. Even if the study didn't help her, she says: "It would help the doctors out so they would know more about my arthritis and they could help other kids with it."

Under TREAT, all children receive weekly methotrexate shots. In addition, they're randomly assigned to one of two groups. One group will also receive etanercept (*Enbrel*) and oral prednisolone. The second group will appear to be receiving the same regimen, but the etanercept and the prednisolone will actually be placebos.

The children and families involved are blinded to which medications they're receiving, although nothing prevents them from guessing. Danielle, Daina's mother, believes her daughter did receive the placebos because she didn't experience much relief. After four months, Daina was assessed to be only 30 percent better.

TREAT offers children and their parents another option, called open-label. After four months on the first medication regimen, children who aren't at least 70 percent better are offered the option to take etanercept and prednisolone. (They still won't know what they originally received.) Daina accepted and, within a week or so, her mother started noticing the difference. Her penmanship had improved, she could carry her baby sister and she no longer walked downstairs clutching the railing with both hands. "Now she zooms up and down them," Danielle says. "I've got my daughter back."

> "It would help the doctors... and they could help other kids."

otherwise designed to match the real drug—instead of the medication being studied.

But unlike research in adults, in which the placebo could be the only treatment, additional protective steps are taken in research involving children. Typically, children involved in research trials will receive some base-line treatment. For example, in the TREAT trial (short for Trial of Early Aggresive Drug Therapy in Juvenile Idiopathic Arthritis), all children participating are receiving methotrexate shots at the minimum. Another protective approach—also available in the TREAT trial—is to offer a multiphase study. In the first phase, the treatment includes a placebo. But the next phase is open-label. That means if your child doesn't meet certain criteria for improvement, you will be given the option to switch her to the medication being studied.

To learn more about clinical trials and what's currently available, there's a wealth of information online. One good place to start is the National Institutes of Health site, **www.clinicaltrials.gov**; it breaks down research trials by medical condition. A Web site more specific to juvenile arthritis is run by the Childhood Arthritis and Rheumatology Research Alliance (CARRA) at **www.carragroup.org**. Click on "current studies" to learn what trial options are available for JIA, lupus and other rheumatic diseases.

Medication Bottom Line

Although it may seem tempting some days, skipping medication isn't an option. True, juvenile arthritis isn't as immediately life-threatening as some childhood diseases, such as Type 1 (juvenile) diabetes. But giving yourself and your child a free pass sends the wrong message if you're trying to teach the importance of strict medication management.

Sometimes you'll be advised by your child's doctor to skip a dose or two because of medical reasons; your child might be battling the flu or another serious infection. But think twice before allowing your child to jettison a dose because of the daily stresses of life, whether it's the logistics of a family trip or the sadness of that first romantic break up.

In the end, no single shot or pill will stem the tide of inflammation. But finding the right combination of medications, and taking them day after day, will do more than help shield your child's joints from the damaging effects of inflammation. It will buy her crucial time, allowing researchers to develop, refine and expand the arsenal of drug interventions. ●

. . . .

CHAPTER EIGHT

Special Considerations: The Eyes, Jaw and Stature

Arthritis inflammation may weaken parts of the body in ways that can be difficult to detect, particularly at first. Shortly after diagnosis, your child may be more prone to complaining about discomfort in the joints that move her limbs—knees, ankles, wrists and so on. But your child's other joints and body parts can be equally vulnerable, so pay close attention.

For instance, arthritis can inflict inflammatory damage on a critical joint in the jaw, called the temporomandibular joint, or TMJ. The result can be pain, stiffness, swelling and even growth changes. If the damage progresses too far, your child may find it difficult to chew, brush her teeth or yawn. At the same time, her vision also can be threatened if worrisome white blood cells infiltrate the eye itself. This kind of eye inflammation can be sneaky, frequently with no pain or other symptoms.

With both complications, though, early diagnosis and intervention can make all the difference. Frequent checkups can detect the cells before they erode your child's vision. And clicking or other noisy movements in the jaw can signal more trouble to come. When identified early enough, your child may need only relatively minor treatment—such as eye drops or jaw protection techniques—along with her regular arthritis medication to fore-stall further damage.

Protecting Your Child's Eyes

Eye inflammation that is experienced by children with JIA is frequently called uveitis because it affects a portion or all of the uveal tract, a layer just under the white part of the eye. For reasons that are unclear, the area may become inflamed and the eye can develop symptoms, such as redness or pain. Or, in many children with some types of JIA, uveitis may be chronic but symptom-free, making it difficult for you to detect as a parent. That is why regular eye exams are extremely important for your child.

PERSONAL ESSAY

SEEING THE WORLD THROUGH UVEITIS
Holland Marrone's Essay

JRA has affected me my whole life. I don't know life without it. I guess it began in my right foot and moved up to my right knee. It has now moved to my left knee, too. I've never been able to run and play sports as well as other kids. When I do run, my right knee swells and I can't bend it very well. Sometimes it feels as if my knee's going to pop open from all the pressure.

Then the disease spread to my eye. When my eye flares, my head feels like it's going to explode. The headaches are usually right above my eyes. They get sensitive to the light and my left eye gets very blood shot. There is so much pressure put on my brain that I can't laugh, look at bright things, or even cough.

To ease the pain, I use ice packs, make my bedroom very dark and take extra medication. Sometimes I have to take my glasses off and go to sleep for a few hours. I use eye drops almost every day, but only in my left eye. Sometimes I don't have any eye problems at all, but I still have to see my eye doctor every three months. Mom says we can never miss that appointment.

I know I will have to take medication for the rest of my life. Since I've been on [adalimumab] *Humira*, my eye problems haven't been as bad and I am able to enjoy more play time with my friends. Life comes at you fast, so I've learned to enjoy it the way it is and try to live and love life.

—*Holland Marrone is 14 years old and lives near Detroit.*

In kids with JIA, significant eye damage can unfold undetected. One pediatric rheumatologist describes a particularly bad example, a fourth-grade boy with arthritis who'd gone a year and a half without an eye exam. His parents insisted on the exam after he broke his glasses. The optometrist at the eyeglasses store couldn't even see into one of the boy's eyes because of the scarring, but the boy hadn't complained of any vision difficulties.

Besides the frequent lack of symptoms, chronic uveitis is tricky for a number of other reasons. The progression and severity of the eye inflammation may likely mirror your child's joint inflammation. However, your child may have limited inflammation in the joints, but a severe case of uveitis (or the other way around). Chronic uveitis may also break other patterns. Although it typically develops in young children within a few years of diagnosis, eye inflammation also has emerged more than a decade after arthritis was diagnosed.

But when identified and treated early, uveitis is one of medicine's prevention success stories. Research studies have demonstrated that early intervention can halt, or at least greatly suppress, the inflammatory process and thus help prevent long-term problems, including cataracts, glaucoma and blindness.

ASSESSING RELATIVE EYE RISK: Most uveitis cases associated with JIA occur within the first four years of arthritis onset. Researchers break uveitis into several types, with specific names depending on which part of the eye is involved. Children with common types of JIA, such as oligoarthritis (pauciarticular) or polyarthritis, are usually diagnosed with anterior uveitis, inflammation that involves the front of the eye. The technical term, less commonly used outside of medical circles, is iridocyclitis.

Traditionally, this chronic form of inflammation was believed to be largely confined to young children (particularly young girls) with arthritis in a limited number of joints, called oligoarthritis under the JIA criteria. In recent years, though, there's been a heightened awareness that the inflammation also can a strike

....

EYES: RISKY
MEDICATIONS
A few juvenile arthritis medications can be potentially risky for the eyes and thus require additional monitoring. Two to watch out for:

Corticosteroids: This class of drugs, which includes prednisone, can lead to cataracts over time. Adults are considered more vulnerable than children, but regular checks are still recommended.

Hydroxychloroquine (Plaquenil): Over time, this anti-malarial drug can lead to difficulties in distinguishing the color red. Annual exams can screen for any changes in sharpness of vision or color-related problems.

a child with arthritis in a few more joints, technically classified with having polyarthritis.

Another potential red flag is your child's results on a blood test for antinuclear antibodies, known as the ANA test. If your child tests positive for ANA, she will be scheduled for more frequent eye checks, in accordance with the screening guidelines set by the American Academy of Pediatrics. (*See box below.*) Uveitis also can develop in a child who tests negative for the antibody marker.

Still, there are some basic benchmarks. A majority of children develop chronic eye inflammation within seven years after the autoimmune disease is diagnosed; the risk of uveitis is greatest within the first two years. The average age of diagnosis is between 6 and 8 years. Both eyes are likely to be affected.

Although chronic (and potentially symptomless) uveitis is more common in children with JIA, an acute form also can emerge with a sudden onset of symptoms. Your child might complain of pain, redness or light sensitivity. That form is more commonly identified in children who test

....

UVEITIS SCREENING GUIDELINES

The American Academy of Pediatrics (AAP) provides guidelines on screening for uveitis for juvenile rheumatoid arthritis. Children who test positive for antinuclear antibodies are considered more vulnerable. But all children with pauciarticular, polyarticular or systemic arthritis should be regularly checked.

To simplify the complex screening guidelines, the physicians at the University of Minnesota provide a break down of relative risk:

HIGHER RISK Any child with the oligoarticular (pauciarticular) or polyarticular form of arthritis who tests

positive for antinuclear antibody (ANA) and is younger than age 7 when the disease develops.
Recommendation: Should have a slit-lamp eye exam every three months for the first four years. For the next three years, she should be checked every six months and annually after that.

MIDDLE RISK Any child with oligoarticular (pauciarticular) or polyarticular arthritis who tests negative for ANA and is younger than age 7 when the disease develops. Or, a child who tests positive for ANA, but is 7 years or older at disease onset.

Recommendation: Should have a slit-lamp exam every six months for the first four years, followed by annual screenings.

LOWER RISK Any child with oligoarticular (pauciarticular) or polyarticular arthritis who tests negative for ANA and is 7 years or older when the autoimmune disease is diagnosed. Or, any patients with systemic arthritis.
Recommendation: Should have a slit-lamp eye examination annually.

If your child has another form of arthritis not covered in the AAP guidelines, be sure to check with your child's rheumatologist for recommendations.

positive for HLA-B27, the genetic marker commonly associated with the spondyloarthropathies, such as juvenile ankylosing spondylitis.

DIAGNOSIS AND TREATMENT: It is important that you arrange for your child to see an ophthalmologist, not an optometrist, or that if you do go to an optometrist for a vision test make sure to tell this professional your child has JIA because they may need to allot enough time for tests.

To diagnose uveitis, the ophthalmologist will use a slit lamp exam. The test, quick and painless despite its odd-sounding name, involves using a microscope to get a three-dimensional view of your child's eye to see any signs of active inflammation. The test, which usually takes five to 10 minutes, is conducted by shining a narrow beam of strong light from the slit lamp into your child's eye while the eye doctor uses a microscope to scrutinize its structure and functioning.

The doctor will search for individual white blood cells floating in the eye, which shouldn't be there. If they're present, the doctor will count them. At the same time, the doctor will look for signs of scarring. For example, if the eye's pupil doesn't constrict normally when the light shines on it, that might indicate that scar tissue is hampering its movement.

Once uveitis is diagnosed, the doctor will probably begin some type of steroid treatment to bring the inflammation under control as quickly as possible. Anti-inflammatory steroid eye drops are considered to be the cornerstone of initial treatment. Your child also may be briefly prescribed steroid pills or an injection delivered to the region of the eye. Regular appointments with the ophthalmologist will be necessary, as well.

If the steroids alone aren't sufficient to beat back the inflammation, your child's doctor may take a two-pronged approach, combining the eye drops with a medication that fights inflammation throughout the body, such as an NSAID, methotrexate or a biologic. To date, adalimumab (*Humira*) and infliximab (*Remicade*) appear to be the most effective biologics at combating uveitis.

The goal is to eliminate any signs of inflammation, without requiring the ongoing use of steroids. Even subtle, smoldering disease can elevate the risk of long-term effects, but aggressive treatment can make a difference in terms of long-term vision problems.

A 2007 study found that of 142 children diagnosed with uveitis, 53 developed at least one vision-related complication. Cataracts were seen most frequently and glaucoma also was relatively common. Even so, more than 90 percent of the children with uveitis had normal vision at their last follow-up visit, and fewer than 6 percent were blind.

Guarding the Jaw

As inflammation attacks your child's joints, one potential and pivotal sore spot is the temporomandibular joint (TMJ). All of us have these two crucial hinges that connect the lower jaw bone to the temporal bone on the side of the skull. They are sophisticated joints, allowing your child to not only open and close her mouth, but also move her jaw back and forth and from side to side. As a result, she may rely on these joints hundreds of times each day for numerous basic activities: eating, yawning, tooth brushing, talking.

Unfortunately, your child also may be vulnerable to inflammatory damage in the TMJ. The most common symptom, identified in nearly one-third of patients, is restricted ability to open the mouth. This problem can affect your child's speech, chewing and other important daily activities—and cause her embarrassment as well.

ARTHRITIS AND TMJ: The pain involved in arthritis of the jaw can stem from several sources. It may be directly related to the arthritis itself or to the displacement of the cartilage that's designed to cushion the joint, allowing it to open or close smoothly. Pain also can result from the strain placed on the muscles supporting the temporomandibular joint. Those muscles may tighten in an effort to prevent the jaw from moving. But those tightened muscles can trigger some of their own painful symptoms, such as spasms and the restriction of normal jaw motion.

Besides causing pain, arthritis can lead to degenerative changes in the jaw, affecting how the teeth meet and creating other health issues. Once jaw damage progresses to a certain extent, alignment difficulties can become noticeable. When both joints are involved, the chin can recede, affecting your child's profile. If one joint is more affected than another, a crooked jaw can be the result.

Along with the cosmetic issues, jaw alignment difficulties can make it difficult to bite into food—say an apple—or chew. A poorly aligned jaw also can be associated with obstructive sleep apnea. Sometimes the joint damage can persist undetected for years and, in rare instances, the detection of jaw problems by a dental specialist may be the first step toward diagnosing arthritis elsewhere in the body.

So when should your child see a dental specialist? That will be up to your child's rheumatologist, who should be checking her jaw as part of a regular joint exam. Be sure to alert your physician, however, if your child develops a clicking or grating/grinding sound when she opens her mouth. Also, look for even subtle changes in her jaw's alignment or any difficulties in chewing or stretching her jaw wide.

EASY LIFESTYLE CHANGES: Surgery, as with other arthritis-related complications, is far less common these days for treatment of TMJ problems. Depending on the severity of your child's TMJ symptoms, the dental specialist may prescribe medication—in coordination with your child's rheumatologist—and exercises. But the cornerstone of reducing discomfort is changing some basic lifestyle habits.

The goal is to reduce, as much as possible, the strain on those two critical joints. Try to discourage your child from resting her jaw on her hand while surfing the computer or when bored in class. Keep her away, as much as possible, from chewing gum and other chewy treats, such as caramels or licorice. That constant chewing action places a lot of strain on those joints.

Don't assume, however, your child should be sentenced to a diet of pureed food. Like all her joints, it's important that she keeps her jaw muscles and joints flexible and strong. Instead, cut your child's food in very small bites so she can put a little piece on each side of her mouth. That way, she's eating slowly and working both joints and won't be tempted to compensate for a sore side by relying too much on the opposite side.

Above all, teach her not to clench her teeth. What's clenching? You may be surprised to learn that lightly touching teeth are considered clenched. The pumping action of the jaw closing and opening is needed to circulate the synovial fluid. When your child holds her teeth together, even lightly, that shuts down the supply of vital joint nourishment.

Instead, your child should rest her tongue gently against the roof of her mouth, in the same position she uses to make a "clucking" sound. That should be her relaxed position. It's a potentially difficult habit to implement, but one that could protect her temporomandibular joints over the long haul.

Along with lifestyle changes, your child may find that heat or cold treatments provide some temporary pain relief. Heat a wet towel in a microwave, wrap it around a gel pack and apply to the joint for 15 to 20 minutes to allow the heat to penetrate to the muscles and joint. Or, your child can try a cold treatment by applying a cold gel pack or rubbing an ice cube on the joint. Expect the area to first burn and then go numb; stop when it goes numb. Your child should use the approach that works best for her.

Exercises also can be beneficial. Exactly which ones will depend upon your child's function difficulties. Exercises can be used to rotate the jaw, relax the tightened muscles around the inflamed joint or stretch the joint itself.

BEYOND SELF-CARE: If lifestyle changes and self-care don't provide adequate relief, members of your child's medical team will be able to provide additional options. One is the use of a dental appliance. A variety are available that can be used to either protect the joint at night or help to reposition it over time.

As for medications, your child's dental specialist will likely coordinate with her rheumatologist. Steroid injections are one strategy. The last resort would be some type of surgical procedure to help reduce inflammation or realign the jaw.

One less invasive surgical approach is a procedure called arthrocentesis, in which the surgeon injects the joint with local anesthetic and fluid to help flush out inflamed fluids. Steroids may be injected at the same time.

Jaw alignment problems also may be tackled by a surgical procedure to cut and reposition the jawbone, holding it in place with screws. Replacement of the temporomandibular joint can be performed, although it's considered a last resort and is quite rare. In the event total replacement becomes necessary, the surgeon may replace your child's joint with a procedure using bone and cartilage from one of your child's own ribs or use an artificial joint.

Growth Issues: Coming Up Short

Arthritis, or the related treatment, may shave some inches off your child's height, either temporarily or over the long haul. The risk can vary significantly, depending upon your child's diagnosis, treatment and nutritional health.

Oligoarticular arthritis (previously called pauciarticular) is less likely to suppress growth overall, although it may impact specific joints. Children with polyarticular or systemic diagnoses are considered more vulnerable. Those children with systemic arthritis potentially face a two-fold risk. To treat the disease, your child may be prescribed corticosteroids, an effective intervention with the potential side effect of stunting growth.

Other influences also can affect stature. Your child may be inadequately nourished, either because of joint pain in the jaw or medication side effects, such as nausea. Food also can become a tool of rebellion. Weary of all the arthritis-related rules, your child may fight over what's on her plate as something she can control.

Will your child always be shorter than average? A lot of variables come into play, including the age at which your child's arthritis was diagnosed, its overall severity and the length of time on steroids. Treatment and diagnosis around puberty can have a greater ripple effect, given the growth spurt in those years. The loss of physical stature can be challenging amid the rough and tumble world of growing up. This may be especially true for boys, since physical size and prowess can play a greater role in play and friendships.

To ease some of those emotional speed bumps, talk up your child's strengths, ones that can't be measured with a ruler. You might delay your child's enrollment in school by a year, so she can accumulate confidence. And, as the years unfold, make sure that others treat your child based on her emotional age and maturity, rather than physical stature. ●

....

CHAPTER NINE

Surgical Options: Procedures and Considerations

In the last two decades, surgery has been pushed to the back burner of juvenile arthritis treatment. Thanks to the emergence and more aggressive use of powerful drugs, your child faces a much lower risk of developing joint damage that's substantial enough to require some type of surgical intervention.

By combining medication with other tools, your child's joints can be protected for a longer period of time and functioning challenges may be reduced or, ideally, eliminated. Drugs aren't the only method for alleviating juvenile arthritis symptoms and avoiding surgery. For example, regular stretching and exercise can help prevent joint contractures, in which healthy connective tissue becomes scarred and inflexible, preventing movement. Assistive devices, such as splints, can be used to support or reposition weakened joints.

Still, surgery and even hospitalization can become unavoidable, typically for one of two reasons. Either an effective medication regimen couldn't be identified to stem the progression of joint damage in your child, or your child may have been diagnosed later in the disease process, after significant inflammatory fallout already has occurred. Surgery, in such cases, can provide relief and restore function.

Seeking Surgical Relief

Over time, inflammation can weaken your child's joints and surrounding tissues in a number of ways. The synovium—the tissue that lines the joint capsule and makes lubrication for your joint—can become inflamed and enlarged, invading and damaging nearby cartilage and bone. Inflammation also can weaken muscles, ligaments and tendons, leaving them unable to support the joint properly.

Surgical procedures can provide several potential benefits, including reducing pain and increasing your child's ability to move and use her joint. Depending on the procedure, an orthopaedic surgeon may remove inflamed tissue or replace an entire joint.

If your child's doctor does recommend surgery, keep in mind that advances in surgical techniques make it more feasible than ever for the procedure to be performed on an outpatient basis, allowing your child to go home for the night. One significant advance is arthroscopy, in which a thin, lighted tube helps the surgeon examine your child's joints or perform some procedures. Through the tube, which is connected to a closed-circuit TV, the surgeon can take a biopsy, remove overgrown synovial lining or

....

BEFORE SURGERY: SOME QUESTIONS TO ASK

You can't ask too many questions if you're contemplating surgery for your child. Don't hesitate to ask the surgeon or pediatric rheumatologist to review any details or risks that you don't understand or that concern you. To help better understand the available options, you also may want to seek out a second opinion.

Here are some questions you may have for your surgeon:

- Can you describe the surgery step-by-step?

- Are there non-surgical treatments that could postpone or eliminate the need for this surgery? How successful might they be?

- How much improvement can my child expect afterwards?

- What are the risks? How likely are those risks?

- What are the risks of my child not having surgery?

- What are the risks of delaying the procedure?

- How long does it take?

- What is your experience doing this type of surgery?

- Is this surgery performed on an outpatient basis or will my child have to be hospitalized?

- What kind of anesthesia will you use? What are the risks of the anesthesia?

- Will my child need to change medications or dosages before or following surgery?

- Can you put me in touch with another family whose child has already had this surgery?

- Will my child require additional surgery after this?

a loose piece of cartilage, or smooth an area that's become rough. (*See box, right.*)

Procedure by Procedure

The following surgical procedures tend to be the most commonly performed on children with arthritis; the more frequent surgical interventions are ranked closer to the top:

EPIPHYSIODESIS: Occasionally arthritis of the knee can cause increased growth in the growth centers of the distal femur (the portion of the upper leg bone closest to the knee) and the proximal tibia (the portion of the lower leg bone closest to the knee), resulting in a discrepancy in leg lengths. Epiphysiodesis is an operation that involves surgically closing one of the growth centers of the longer limb, allowing the shorter limb gradually to catch up in length.

WHY IT'S DONE: To correct a difference in leg lengths that may be caused by accelerated growth of the limb with arthritis.

WHAT ELSE YOU NEED TO KNOW: Epiphysiodesis usually is reserved for children whose anticipated leg-length discrepancy is greater than 2 centimeters (or almost an inch) and who have at least two years of growth remaining. The recovery period is brief, and there are few complications.

JOINT FUSION (ARTHRODESIS): In this procedure, also called bone fusion, the surgeon removes the cartilage from the ends of two bones that form a joint and then positions the bones together and holds them immobile, often with a pin or a rod. Over time, the two bones fuse to form a single solid unit.

WHY IT'S DONE: Arthrodesis can correct joint deformity. It can make the joint more stable, help it bear weight better and relieve pain. It's most likely to be done on specific joints, including the foot/ankle, hand/wrist and spine.

WHAT ELSE YOU NEED TO KNOW: Once a joint is fused, your child will never again be able to bend it. Fusing one joint can place stress on nearby joints and increase the risk of fracture in the bones that are fused.

ARTHROSCOPY: SCOPING OUT ARTHRITIS

One way a doctor can assess arthritis-related damage in your child's joints is by using an arthroscope, a very thin tube with a light at the end. The tube, which is connected to a closed-circuit monitor, can look directly into the joint.

The arthroscope also can be used to take a biopsy or for some procedures, such as removing a loose piece of cartilage, repairing torn cartilage or smoothing a rough joint surface. If surgery can be performed through an arthroscope, it's frequently done on an outpatient basis and recovery is faster and less painful than traditional surgery.

JOINT REPLACEMENT (ARTHROPLASTY): This surgery involves removing a damaged joint and replacing it with an artificial joint made of metal, ceramics and/or plastics.

WHY IT'S DONE: Total joint replacement can often dramatically reduce pain and improve motion, mobility and function. It is usually reserved as the final option for joints that are so severely damaged, painful and stiff that they interfere with the child's functioning and quality of life. The most commonly replaced joint due to JIA is the hip, followed by the knee; rarely is the ankle, wrist or shoulder replaced.

WHAT ELSE YOU NEED TO KNOW: Total joint replacement does have some drawbacks. Replacing joints can stunt growth, and the longevity of prosthetic joints is limited. Most doctors delay the surgery as long as possible for young people. Complications can include premature failure of the synthetic joint or an infection that could potentially necessitate additional surgery.

SYNOVECTOMY: This procedure removes excess synovial tissue. The synovium is normally a thin membrane that lines the joint capsule. With chronic inflammation of this lining (as occurs with juvenile arthritis), it not only produces extra fluid, but grows much thicker and can affect joint structure and function. The vast majority of synovectomies are performed by arthroscopy, a procedure in which surgical tools are inserted through a few small incisions, eliminating the need to open the joint.

WHY IT'S DONE: Synovectomy is designed to limit excess synovial lining that isn't helped by treatments, including intra-articular corticosteroid injections. The procedure most often is done on the knee and occasionally the wrist.

WHAT ELSE YOU NEED TO KNOW: Although synovectomy can relieve pain and swelling, it doesn't stop progression of the disease. In most cases, the synovium grows back in a matter of months or years. For some children, joint pain and swelling are so severe that surgery is worthwhile for even a short period of relief. If it's successful, the procedure can be repeated when the synovium grows back.

The following procedures are performed less often in children:

OSTEOTOMY: Corrects a bone deformity by cutting and repositioning the bone and then resetting it in a better position.

WHY IT'S DONE: Osteotomy is used primarily to fix deformities. By correcting the bone deformities that lead to unusual forces on a joint, and perhaps joint instability and damage, osteotomy also may eliminate or at least delay the need for total joint replacement. The joints it can help include the knee, hip and joints of the foot.

WHAT ELSE YOU SHOULD KNOW: In general, osteotomy is less successful than total joint replacement. Osteotomy can increase stiffness in the hip. Children who have osteotomy to reposition the hip or knee may need total joint replacement later. New bone growth takes several weeks.

SOFT TISSUE RELEASE: In this procedure, a surgeon cuts and repairs tissues that have tightened about a joint (contracture), often due to inflammation of the joint lining.

WHY IT'S DONE: To improve the position of a malaligned joint due to shortening and tightening of the tendons that support it. If not corrected, contractures can cause pain and joint damage and can affect a child's ability to walk and function. Soft tissue release can improve motion and reduce pain. Results tend to be best for the hip and knee, though your child's doctor may recommend it for other joints.

WHAT ELSE YOU NEED TO KNOW: Soft tissue release is most effective when joint destruction is not severe.

Preparing for Hospitalization

If your child's surgery does require a night or two in the hospital, careful planning will help make the process go more smoothly. Although it's important to fill out all of the appropriate forms and complete the pre-operation lab work, some of the most important preparation you can do involves communication—both with the hospital clinicians and your child.

Take time to talk through issues ahead of time with the doctors and nurses, including potential complications relevant to your child's arthritis. Where your child is involved, it's important to answer any questions or concerns she has ahead of time.

You might consider taking a field trip to the hospital. In the process, hopefully you will ferret out some of her worries, and address them, before she's exposed to the unfamiliar walls of a hospital room.

Supporting Your Child

When you talk to your child, explain in simple language why she's having the surgery and what will happen during her hospital stay. Be very specific. Will the surgery help her knee or hip so she'll be able to move better? Ask your child to repeat back her understanding. That will give you an opportunity to address any misconceptions or clarify any details, so surprises will be minimized.

Make sure your child knows that the hospital isn't punishment for anything she's done. Be sure to describe what will happen during the surgery itself, including anesthesia, if it will be required. Explain that she will be asleep during the surgery and will wake up later. Encourage your child to express her fears. Does she dread anything in particular? If needles are her biggest worry, suggest that she might want to practice giving a shot to a stuffed animal.

Recognize, if appropriate, that there will be unpleasant parts. Try not to hold back any information; your child can sense if you are dodging or withholding. If you can't answer a particular question, tell her that you don't know and that you'll find out the details.

Among other measures that might help make your child feel more "at home" away from her own bed:

• Ask hospital clinicians to use your child's nickname, if that's how she's known.

• If permitted, pack some of your child's favorite things, such as a blanket, pajamas, toy, stuffed animal, books and so on. An older child might want magazines and her favorite music.

• Explain when you'll be at the hospital and when you'll be away, to ease fears of separation. Urge friends and family to visit often.

• Take advantage of any hospital programs for children. For example, the hospital may permit your child to visit the operating room ahead of time.

Assisting the Clinicians

Just as you prepare your child, it's also important to communicate with the hospital's nurses and doctors. Share any important details of your child's medical history, such as past experience with medications, bed rest, splinting or exercise. Emphasize any problems that might interfere with her treatment or recovery. For example, if your child will require general anesthesia for surgery, and her neck mobility is limited, let the anesthesiologist or nurse anesthetist know so they don't inadvertently force her neck farther than its usual range of motion.

Once your child is in the hospital, you'll need to continue acting as her advocate. Concerned about some aspect of your child's care? Talk to a nurse or a doctor rather than keeping those worries to yourself. But also take the time to compliment those clinicians who make an extra effort amid their busy days. Your feedback will help them improve their treatment practices, particularly if they have limited experience caring for a child with arthritis.

And don't forget to take good care of yourself. Get as much sleep as you can and eat right. Above all, stay calm. A clear head will help you better communicate with your child's doctors if anything unexpected should occur. Your confidence also will help soothe any nagging fears your child may harbor. If you are snappish or nervous around your child in the hospital room, she may lose confidence in the procedure's positive outcome. ●

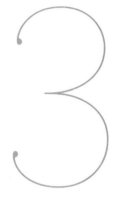

Living With Juvenile Arthritis

In this section, we'll move past medical treatment to discuss other issues that shape your child's life and affect her well-being. We'll examine some of the causes of pain, and we'll talk about basic body mechanics and small adjustments that may improve your child's ability to perform everyday tasks. We'll look at ways to boost your child's physical activity, including examples of specific exercises to maintain your child's flexibility. Then, we'll delve into the emotional aspects of living with arthritis, both for your child and the rest of your family.

CHAPTER TEN

Understanding Pain: Causes and Interventions

Pain, if left untreated, can become one of the most confusing and difficult symptoms to resolve when raising a child with juvenile arthritis. It's even trickier to unravel the underlying causes. The sensations typically described as pain are multifaceted, with physical and psychological components. Researchers have coined the term "the pain puzzle" to depict the interlocking elements that result in the uncomfortable sensations we label as pain.

Although pain is typically not the initial complaint of children when diagnosed with arthritis, recent studies indicate that most children diagnosed with arthritis do report some mild to moderate pain. At least one-fourth describe their pain symptoms as moderate to severe, using such words as aching, sharp, burning and uncomfortable.

The physical signs of pain may be easy to spot. Your child's discomfort may stem from unresolved inflammation that causes swelling, warmth and, occasionally, redness. In cases of more severe disease, the pain can result from the damage to and erosion of the joints themselves. Pain also can reverberate in other ways. Your child may be repositioning her body in an effort to avoid pain, such as by keeping an elbow bent against one side. As a result, the nearby muscles may tighten and ache as they try to protect against further joint pain.

Other influences—both internal and external—can aggravate pain, or at least how your child experiences it. Those include your child's level of fatigue, physical conditioning and state of mind, along with your own modeling behaviors and interactions as a parent. Some children may simply be more sensitive to pain than others.

A chicken-and-egg situation can develop. For example, it can become difficult to tell whether the pain causes fatigue or if fatigue is worsening the pain. It is also important to know that nonphysical influences can aggravate pain, or at least how your child experiences it.

Doctors do not necessarily agree on the best treatment approach to the pain puzzle—especially in children. In the years ahead, you may encounter a mixed bag of feedback. In particular, doctors may adhere to differing philosophies regarding the roles of cognitive approaches, such as positive thinking, versus pain medication. They also may differ on other subjects, including the degree to which you should adopt a tough-love mindset, that is, pushing your child to stay active in school and elsewhere despite ongoing discomfort.

Disagreements notwithstanding, doctors typically agree that you should follow certain key steps for relieving your child's pain. Above all, make sure your child is prescribed—and is regularly taking—an effective arthritis medication regimen that can eliminate as much disease activity as feasible. Be sure to rule out depression, fatigue and other pain promoters. Whenever possible, your child should attempt mental strategies and other nonpharmaceutical interventions, such as deep relaxation, massage and heat treatments, before adding pain pills. To that end, you as a parent have significant influence to assist or impede your child's pain relief.

Physical Nature of Pain

To assemble the pieces of the pain puzzle, it's important to first understand some of the basic physical wiring that triggers the body's alarm system, causing pain. Pain is typically divided into two types—acute and chronic. Acute pain usually stems from a specific cause, such as inflammation or injury to the tissues. In some situations, acute pain can be protective. When your child brushes against a hot stove, nerves send red-alert signals to the brain with such speed that she jumps back before even realizing it. In juvenile arthritis, pain also can serve a highly protective role.

PERSONAL ESSAY

PUSHING THROUGH PAIN
Trina VerSteeg Wilcox's Essay

I look down at my puffy hand and scowl at my red, achy joints. Even I wonder how I can run a marathon, yet opening a soda can get the best of me. I need to use my "tab grabber" and that aggravates me. Years ago, in the presence of company, I might have played the vanity card and pretended that my nails had just been manicured before requesting assistance to open a soda. As I get older and more confident, it's easier to ask for help because I see that even people without arthritis often need help.

Sometimes, though, I do feel like a master of disguise. I don't want people to see that I'm in pain. So I find ways to laugh about it or to change the subject. One day my feet were hurting and someone asked in a rather loud voice, "Are you limping?" I had to think quickly—I didn't feel like explaining why my feet hurt. "I hope not," I replied. "If so, I better drop these shoes in the trash and call it a day!" I half smiled and quickly went on my way, careful not to limp.

I've been told by doctors that I have a high threshold for pain. Therefore, I often will not even realize that I am having an extra pain-filled day until I notice I'm being grumpy toward people or getting down on myself.

One of the best ways I keep pain at bay is with exercise. It keeps me limber and allows me to clear my mind. Getting aggravated perpetuates pain. It is comforting for me to be around family and friends who recognize when I need assistance, give me a bit of help (just as I would for them), and then move on with life. When people do not make a big deal about providing me assistance, it reminds me how everybody needs help sometimes, and it is nothing to be ashamed of.

Pain medication also can be very helpful. It is not easy for me to admit that I need to take medication to feel better, since I strive for a very healthy lifestyle. However, all things in moderation and I believe that if you feel better then you will be happier. And being happy is the best life extender you can come to know.

> "I do feel like a master of disguise. I don't want people to see that I'm in pain."

—*Trina VerSteeg Wilcox, age 31, has completed six marathons. She was diagnosed with juvenile arthritis at age 6.*

An acutely swollen joint emits its own pain signal—alerting your child to take a break and stop using that joint.

Acute pain, which tends to develop suddenly, can be diagnosed and treated. Acute pain is a finite thing—it lasts for a short time, then subsides. Chronic pain is more likely to persist over an extended period of time, and pain sensations can be heightened by environmental and psychological influences.

EASING PAIN: JOINT BY JOINT

Depending upon the joint involved, pain can change the way your child moves. A child with neck pain may be unable to look up, while another child with elbow or wrist pain may position joints differently, making it harder or even impossible—over time—to fully straighten them.

The solutions may be just as varied and include splints, therapeutic exercises or more informal daily modifications. A head-to-toe guide:

NECK: A child with neck pain may struggle to look up or turn her head sideways. She'll compensate by moving her shoulders or entire body rather than twisting her neck. Quite often, the surrounding muscles will hurt as much as the joints themselves.
SOME SOLUTIONS: Place moist heat on her muscles to help them relax. Sleeping with a cervical pillow—or no pillow at all—also helps to alleviate neck pain. Elevate the television to encourage motion in the neck. Range-of-motion exercises also can help prevent loss of motion and decrease pain.

JAW: The temporomandibular joint can be a frequent source of discomfort, making it painful to bite into a thick sandwich or an apple. Jaw pain is common on the side of the face or just in front of the ear.
SOME SOLUTIONS: When your child experiences jaw pain, serve softer foods that require less force to eat, cut food into small bites and have her avoid chewing gum. Consult your child's physical therapist about exercises that may relieve pain.

ELBOW: A child with elbow pain is more likely to keep the joint bent, holding it close to the body. It's important to encourage your child to straighten her elbow, as she may lose the ability to do so over time if she continues to hold it in a protective position. Over time, holding any joint in a bent position may cause the muscles on that side to shorten.
SOME SOLUTIONS: Try activities and exercises that encourage straightening, such as pushing away light objects or "pushing" pretend objects up to the ceiling.

WRIST: A child with wrist pain typically holds her wrist curled in her lap. Raising it or making a fist becomes problematic.
SOME SOLUTIONS: Therapists work on strengthening the muscles on the back and side of the arm. Splints are commonly

How pain occurs in the body and how we experience it is something researchers are still striving to understand. They believe that brain chemicals—also called neurotransmitters—play a role by helping to transmit the sensations of pain between cells in the brain and the spinal cord. Some of those chemicals may stimulate mild pain, whereas others influence stronger pain sensations. At the same time, the brain attempts to alleviate pain

used. A functional wrist splint may help your child perform daily tasks with less pain. Resting splints at night provide extra support and prevent deformity.

FINGERS: Children with finger pain may be unable to pick up small objects or have trouble writing because they tend to keep their fingers in a curled position.
SOME SOLUTIONS: To ease pain, your child should use large crayons or pencils, or those with soft grip covers. An older child may prefer to type on a computer. Another option is to use a gel-type pen with ink that flows easily, to reduce resistance or dragging as she writes. To strengthen your child's fingers, have her use play-dough, putty or a squishy ball.

HIP: When children have hip involvement, the extensor muscles become weaker than the opposing flexor muscles, pulling the hip forward so it becomes curled up.
SOME SOLUTIONS: While watching television or reading, your child can lie on her stomach to stretch hips into extension after sitting flexed all day at school.

KNEE: Knee involvement is common in arthritis. Once it becomes difficult

to straighten the knee, your child may walk with a limp. Parents will notice that smaller children no longer can squat.
SOME SOLUTIONS: When experiencing knee pain, your child should rest with the knee straight and the heel propped up. Young children may benefit from wearing a knee extension splint at night to keep the knee extended while sleeping. A therapist can work with your child to strengthen the quadriceps.

ANKLES: Your child's ankle can require some support if it becomes weak and painful.
SOME SOLUTIONS: An in-shoe orthotic can support the structure of the foot to relieve pain when standing and walking. Exercises that stretch the calf muscles and strengthen the muscles that raise the toes can be helpful. Ask your child to perform ankle circles in the bath, using her feet to make letters of the alphabet or to spell secret messages.

FOOT: When your child's foot hurts, pain is usually the worst on the ball of the foot, making it hard to walk or raise the toes.
SOME SOLUTIONS: A small pad, placed just behind the ball of the foot, will relieve pressure on the foot.

through the release of natural pain relievers from the spinal cord, including serotonin and norepinephrine. Endorphins, another natural pain-relieving substance, also can kick in.

Although pain is easy to describe, it's difficult to quantify. No test can measure pain's intensity. And children may describe or reflect their pain in various ways, depending on their age. An older child has both the language and the awareness to pinpoint pain. A younger child, such as a toddler or pre-schooler, may exhibit signs more indirectly—by modifying movements, complaining of being tired, or sitting quietly on a bench while friends play tag.

Studies have shown a clear association between more aggressive disease and stronger pain, but disease activity itself may account for only a portion of your child's reported pain levels. The perception of pain can be highly individual, and your child's may have been altered by years of living with sore, uncomfortable joints. So-called "moderate" pain for your child might be considered "severe" by anyone without arthritis. On the other hand, a few studies have indicated that children with arthritis may actually have developed a lower tolerance for pain, perhaps because of the prolonged assault of painful stimuli.

Your child, even when considered in remission, may continue to complain about lingering pain. How could that be? At this point, there are only theories. One possibility is that the disease, although not identifiable by clinical exam, continues to percolate on a molecular level. Pre-existing joint damage also may play a role. Another possibility is that your child has become sensitized to arthritis pain associated with certain activities or movements, such as walking down stairs, and now instinctually (and incorrectly) attributes any discomfort to arthritis.

Psychological Overlay of Pain

Pain is the result of four interconnecting influences. Beyond the neural impulses themselves, previously described, pain can be shaped and re-shaped by three other elements:

- **FEELINGS:** Anxiety, depression and other emotional stresses can become intertwined with your child's pain sensation. The relationship is by no means absolute. A child in pain doesn't necessarily suffer from depression or vice versa. But there appear to be some crucial links, both emotional and practical. If your child becomes depressed, she may become more aware of ongoing pain. An anxious child may keep her muscles tensed, amplifying existing pain. Conversely, a child in constant pain is less likely to spend time with friends, taking steps toward isolation that can, over time, spiral into depression. Some research also indicates that pain and depression may share some of the same neurochemical pathways, further complicating the equation.

- **THOUGHTS:** How we think about life experiences shapes our perception of them. Pain is no different. Your child's perception of pain can be influenced by her own internal system of beliefs, attitudes and thoughts. Most worrisome is when your child's thought processes become stalled in negative ruts, described as catastrophic thinking. In essence, preoccupation with pain can magnify its effects. Research involving adults with rheumatoid arthritis has revealed that such negative thinking can result in greater pain, depression and functional limitations. It's important to help your child stay positive and hopeful.

- **BEHAVIOR:** Your child's reaction to pain, along with your own, will help mold her coping skills over time. In this piece of the pain puzzle, the parent plays a particularly important role. Bolster your child's coping skills and focus on the things she enjoys and can do rather than letting her dwell on what she cannot do. Search for hobbies, sports or other interests that inspire your child to live beyond those painful joints. As a parent, you also can model good behavior when your own migraines, back aches or other painful symptoms strike.

Does this mean that pain resides only in your child's head? Not at all. Just don't forget the emotional and cognitive components while you're focused on finding the best treatment plan to defuse your child's painful inflammation. Help your child develop good coping skills for when she experiences pain. Pain can seem overwhelming for a child, and she may worry the pain will never go away. Don't let pain define your child's life. She can fight back—and win.

PAIN: TRIGGERS AND TREATMENTS

Pain isn't easy to resolve. What works for another child may not address your child's pain. Here are some potential triggers to avoid, if possible, as well as a number of interventions to try.

SOME TRIGGERS:
- Anxiety
- Depression
- Emotional stress
- Fatigue
- Focusing on pain
- Increased disease activity

SOME TREATMENTS:
- Appropriate exercise
- Heat and cold treatments
- Massage
- Medications
- Humor
- Positive attitude/thoughts
- Relaxation
- Topical pain relievers

Mental Strategies

To help your child, try to get a better sense of her daily pain and personal triggers. Ask your child to keep a diary—or start one yourself for a very young child—that rates each day based on pain and other factors, including mood and any stressors or daily hassles, such as a fight with a friend or a bad grade. Try to spot any trends or associations. One study, which relied on daily diary reports from children with arthritis, identified a significant correlation between stress and mood and increased reports of pain, stiffness and fatigue.

After developing better insight into your child's personal triggers, you can intervene if you see signs that she's heading into a situation that might spark pain. You might notice that your child is not sleeping well or she's slacking off the daily exercises. She might be isolating herself more, pulling away from friends or school commitments.

Are patterns emerging? You can take positive steps to refocus her on the things that boost her energy and spirits. You can reinforce good habits, such as adequate sleep and good nutrition, to prevent your child from inadvertently sapping her mental energy. At the same time, try to help your child keep arthritis in perspective—that arthritis is something she has to manage, but it doesn't define her as a person. When possible, try to maintain an upbeat attitude. Encourage your child to focus on the positive aspects of life rather than to dwell on the pain. In essence, your child must learn to divert that mental dialogue we all have running in our heads to something psychologists describe as positive self-talk. Work with your child to talk to herself in a hopeful, proactive way about what she can do, not what she can't.

You've probably heard your child express plenty of negative thoughts: "I can't stand this. I hate having arthritis. Why did this happen to me?" When your child expresses negative feelings, take note of how that negativity affects her physical symptoms. Does she become more aware of aches and pains? Encourage your child to experiment with substituting more helpful thoughts. Instead of throwing in the towel, your child can work on developing more positive mental tools, including distraction or relaxation techniques.

To assist your child, try jotting down a list of negative statements. Then illustrate how those dispiriting perceptions can be flipped upside down. For example, if your child says, "I don't want to exercise! I'm hurting.

I just want to sit on the couch today," remind her how much better she typically feels after she exercises. Say, "Come on, let's just do a few exercises together. You know how you always feel better after you get moving!" Rewiring negativity is far from easy. Over time it can feel more natural. Such techniques give your child a sense of control by, among other things, teaching problem-solving strategies.

NATURAL RELIEF: DISTRACTION AND RELAXATION

To limit nagging pain, your child can learn to step outside of immediate discomfort through the use of techniques that help to distract and relax.

These techniques, which take time to develop, use the mind to reverse some of the effects of pain on the body, such as tensed muscles and rapid breathing. Or, they can temporarily distract your child.

In general, relaxation techniques are deceptively simple, although they can assume a variety of forms. One method, called progressive muscle relaxation, involves tightening and relaxing various muscle groups in the body, moving slowly up the body from the toes to the head. Your child should hold each muscle as tight as she can for 5 to 10 seconds before allowing it to relax. You can help guide your child through the process: "Tighten all the muscles in your feet. Spread your toes, flex your ankles. Hold it, tighter, tighter, hold it. Now let it go." Encourage your child to picture the tension flowing out as the muscles relax. Slow, deep breaths can help, allowing your child to release all of the air from the lungs and hopefully a bit of pain in the process.

Another technique, called imagery, incorporates pleasant images to transport your child's mind away from aching joints. Audio tapes can be purchased to assist with the process, although they aren't necessary. Your child only needs a quiet setting, such as a bedroom, with the lights dimmed. While your child lies down with eyes closed, you can help direct the imagery process, suggesting that your child focus on a pleasant image. Then encourage your child to place herself there by describing some of the things she can see, smell, hear or touch. Keep in mind that what adults find pleasant and what children find pleasant can be different. A sandy beach may be appropriate for a grown up, but a child's peaceful place may be splashing in the pool and playing on the playground.

For older children, relaxing in the quiet of their room with their favorite music may be all that is needed to achieve relaxation.

With age and confidence, your child can become more adept at performing these techniques. In the process, your child develops a sense of autonomy, by acquiring strategies that can be used at any time, even when a parent isn't nearby.

You, as a parent, can set a positive example as well. Your actions and attitude will speak louder than words. Let your child see how you try—as best as possible—to apply these techniques to your own life. For example, if you tweaked your back lifting a box at work, don't lie on the sofa groaning. Instead say, "My back is bothering me, I'm going to do some stretches, then take a walk around the neighborhood to loosen it up."

Pain Medication: Roles and Pitfalls

In an ideal world, every child's symptoms would be so effectively controlled by arthritis medication that additional pills wouldn't be needed for pain relief. But some stages or phases of the disease can be more painful; among them, a severe flare or significant joint damage that requires surgery.

The decision about prescribing pain medication, and what form it should take, remains a source of ongoing debate among pediatric rheumatologists and other physicians. Some believe that positive thinking, relaxation and other nonpharmaceutical techniques should be sufficient. Others argue that more aggressive pain relief should be pursued. Most physicians fall somewhere along the spectrum in between.

Over-the-counter medication, such as acetaminophen, might be a good first step. But don't allow your child to routinely take extra pills without checking with the doctor. Given all of the other arthritis drugs your child is already prescribed, she may be inadvertently doubling up. Taking extra ibuprofen, for example, when your child is already on a prescription NSAID may increase the risk of stomach, liver or kidney problems. Even too much acetaminophen, for example, could cause some problems with your child's liver tests. Most importantly, increasing pain may signal that your child's arthritis medication is not working as well and the treatment approach should be revaluated.

More aggressive pain medication, such as morphine or oxycodone, require extra care in their use and most likely will be prescribed under a select set of circumstances. Early on, your child may need immediate pain relief while you wait for arthritis medications to kick in or at a later time during a severe flare.

In general, the goal is to carefully tailor the choice and dosage of these powerful medications to achieve needed relief and avoid common side effects, such as nausea, constipation and unwanted sedation during the daytime. Sometimes they provide needed pain relief, and their sedating effects are helpful for getting your child a good night's rest, but at other times, certain drugs may interfere with daytime activities. Alert your child's doctor if the prescription needs to be refilled early or your child appears overly preoccupied with the timing of the next dose.

Unlocking Pain

No single step may be sufficient to unlock your child's pain. It may take time, working with clinicians, to decipher the symptoms and patterns that mark your child's very individual pain process. Once you've minimized your child's pain as much as possible, you can help her better cope with even painful days. Your child will learn—frequently through trial and error—how to protect sore joints and maximize limited energy. (*For more detail, see Chapter 11.*)

You'll have significant work to do as well, as you learn to be sympathetic rather than over-solicitous—a truly delicate balance to strike. Help your child develop techniques, including relaxation and positive self-talk. Making the mental shift won't be easy, but cognitive tools will provide a measure of confidence and control so pain doesn't overshadow your child's life. ●

CHAPTER ELEVEN
....

Daily Life: Improving the Flow

Juvenile arthritis is a part of your child's life now, but that doesn't mean it has to control her life. The strategy is to make the best decisions to protect her joints and, when arthritis presents your child with challenges, to have some tricks in your bag to make daily life easier.

The underlying goal, particularly when your child's disease flares, is conservation: both of your child's scarce energy reserves and the joints themselves. Exercises and therapists, both occupational and physical, can help your child preserve and expand upon her body's strength and flexibility. Catalogs full of adaptive devices and tools, from dressing hooks to jar openers, can facilitate troublesome daily tasks. Just as importantly, your child will learn to recognize and respond to her body's signals of strain and exhaustion.

That learning process, though, will likely unfold in stops and starts, acquired through a sometimes frustrating and laborious process of trial and error for everyone involved. As a parent, you'll learn over time how to assist and when to get out of the way. Like everything else with arthritis, there's a fine line to walk. Coddling won't help anyone, least of all your child. The goal, as your child grows up, is to teach her the best ways to maximize her energy and functioning so she can excel.

Shielding Those Joints

In the initial months after diagnosis, you might consider several sessions with an occupational therapist, a clinician who specializes in helping people better tackle the daily tasks of life. Occupational therapy might not be required on an ongoing basis, thanks to recent improvements in medication. But a therapist's expertise can be very helpful early on, before the full effects of the arthritis medications kick in.

In general, therapists provide instruction on how to use good posture and body positioning to avoid placing undue stress on the neck, hips, knees and other joints. (*See sidebar on page 110 for more on posture.*) To preserve vulnerable joints, in short, your child must learn to use them more wisely.

Take lifting and carrying, as one example. The general advice is that your child should rely on her strongest and largest joints to distribute her weight across a larger surface area. Encourage your child to carry objects, such as a lunch tray, with both hands to avoid stressing a single joint. When possible, items should be held close to the body and your child should keep her palms open, with the fingers straight, so they don't grip. Does the item even need to be lifted? Teach your child that sometimes heavy loads can be slid along the floor instead. Also, there's no shame in seeking out help.

Some movements should be avoided unless absolutely necessary. Gripping objects, for example, places pressure on your child's fingers. Many of the devices we use every day, including combs and pens, rely on that tight gripping action. To prevent pressure from accumulating, simple steps can be taken, such as using pieces of rubberized shelf liner and other materials to build up wider, easier-to-hold handles.

JOINT-PROTECTION TIPS

- Respect pain.
- Avoid stressful positions.
- Change positions frequently.
- Encourage your child to rely primarily on her largest and strongest muscles to perform a task.
- Keep your child's muscles strong and encourage stretches to keep her joints flexible.
- Introduce splints and other assistive devices when helpful.
- Encourage your child to take short breaks to avoid overuse.

Tools for Daily Tasks

Even when your child's inflammation is stabilized, she still can benefit from some basic joint-protection techniques. Morning stiffness is common and can be particularly stressful when time is tight and everyone scrambles to get out the door to work and school.

Frequently, only a slight modification in routine or a simple device—such as adding loops to clothing zippers—can make the logistics of grooming and eating go more smoothly. **Consider a few of the ideas below:**

BATHING AND GROOMING: Getting up in the morning and into the bathroom can be a chore for any child. Dealing with sore joints and fatigue after a bad night's sleep can make it even harder. **Here are some tips to ease the process:**

- Rouse your child sufficiently early that she can get ready for the day without feeling rushed.
- Suggest a morning bath or shower to decrease morning stiffness. You can warm up the water, so it's ready when your child hits the bathroom.
- Line the tub with a non-slip mat to help prevent falls. Other devices, such as a grab bar next to the tub or toilet, also may be helpful.
- Place a bench in the back of the tub to allow your child to sit while showering.
- Show your child how the toothpaste can be squeezed with the palm of

GETTING AN ASSIST: SPLINTS AND SHOE INSERTS

Splints or shoe inserts provide one alternative if your child's joints need more support or have become bent in the wrong direction.

Depending on how they're designed and used, splints can help stretch the joint back to its correct position or encourage it to remain in a specific position. Orthotics or shoe inserts can help your child compensate for differences in leg length or joint alignment.

Splints, manufactured from a variety of materials, are usually customized to your child's joint and body mechanics challenges. Commonly used splints include those worn on the knee or the wrist.

Resting splints help support inflamed joints with the goal of retaining the correct position and preventing deformities. The wrist, for example, may be splinted during the night. A resting splint may be removed periodically so your child can exercise the joint.

Other devices, called functional splints, can support and ease stress on your child's joint during school and other daily activities. Sometimes the splint may be specifically designed to help your child stretch her muscles while walking or moving through the day. Shoe inserts also can play a functional role by correcting body alignment or easing pain.

PERFECTING YOUR CHILD'S POSTURE

Your child's body alignment, or posture, can make or break the strain placed on joints over the course of a day. Unfortunately, your child likely doesn't have many peer role models; too many children slump over their school desks or the computer keyboard.

Learning how to stand, sit or lie correctly will likely require some additional coaching. For some guidance, take a look at the figures and key points below.

STANDING: Suggest that your child pictures a straight line that runs through her body, connecting her ears, shoulders, hips and knees—all the way down to the feet. Your child should not lock the knees, but allow them to bend slightly. When standing for prolonged periods becomes painful, your child can lean against a wall or put one foot on a low stool to ease strain on the back.

SITTING: At all times, your child's feet should be touching the ground or a footrest. Her hips, knees and ankles should be positioned at a 90-degree angle. To achieve the correct position, your child may require an adjustable chair. Avoid chairs with a soft or "sling" seat. To support the lower back, a towel or pillow can be inserted behind the back.

LYING DOWN: Supporting your child's neck is key to avoid strain on those muscles. Try a cervical (neck) pillow or roll up a towel and place it behind her neck. Avoid placing pillows beneath your child's knees; the muscles can contract, making it difficult to later straighten them.

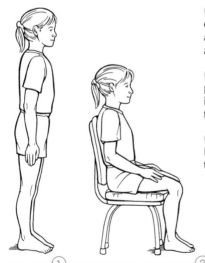

① Correct Standing Posture: The head and shoulders are back, and the chest is lifted. The buttocks are tucked under. The toes are pointed straight ahead with feet slightly apart.

② Correct Sitting Posture: The chair should support the back. The head and back are straight and in line with each other. The feet are placed firmly on the floor.

③ Correct Reclining Posture: Use a firm mattress. Hold arms and legs straight. Use a pillow that is contoured to support your child's head.

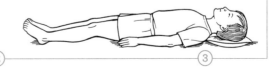

① ② ③

the hand, without straining sore fingers. Another alternative: Purchase a pump bottle of toothpaste.

- Buy an electric toothbrush, which usually has a wider handle than a standard one.
- Help your child find a flattering wash-and-wear hair style. Barring that, purchase a lightweight hair dryer.

DRESSING: Getting dressed is a lot easier when baggy clothes and slip-on shoes, like clogs, are the fashion. But any clothing trend can be modified to meet your child's needs. If cowboy boots are the rage, one option might be to purchase ropers, which have less pointy toes and a lower heel. **Here are some other ideas:**

- To streamline the morning routine, ask your child to choose clothes the night before and lay them out.
- Buy clothes that are easy to pull on and take off. Clothes with snaps or hook-and-loop fasteners are typically easier than buttons.
- Add loops to zippers to make pulling easier.
- To soothe joints and ease morning stiffness, warm clothes in the dryer before pulling them on.
- Look for Velcro-fastening if shoe laces are an issue.
- A long-handled shoehorn can help your child pull on shoes. A dressing stick can assist with clothes.

EATING: Lighter-weight styles of dishes and utensils can be purchased to serve the entire family so your child doesn't feel singled out. Other modifications, such as adjusting how your child holds a cup, also can simplify eating. **Try these:**

- Purchase knives, forks and other utensils with wider handles, so your child finds them easier to grasp.
- Look for light-weight dishes, including mugs or cups with large handles.
- Teach your child to use both hands to grasp a cup or glass, spreading her fingers all the way around.
- If holding a cup is difficult, your child may prefer to use a flexible straw.
- To keep your child's dishes in place at the table, you may consider using rubberized shelf liner material as a placemat.

AROUND THE HOUSE: Walk around your house, spotting potential obstacles from your child's perspective. A doorknob may feel more like a locked door on days your child's wrist or hand is aching. **Consider these tips:**

- To build up hard-to-grasp household items, buy a bag of foam hair rollers. Once you remove the plastic center, you can slide the remaining foam tube over the handle.
- Rubber grips can be slid onto slippery fixtures, such as door knobs and bathroom faucet handles.
- Where feasible, replace door knobs with levers. Bar-style handles might be easier for your child than cabinet knobs.
- Invest in a roll of rubbery shelf-liner material. By cutting it into squares, you can provide some extra leverage for your child, for everything from gripping a door knob to building up the handle of a tool.

Diet and Nutrition

As you strive to support your child's joints, don't forget about the body's first building block: good nutrition. Arthritis emerges during the growing years, when eating nutrient-rich food is crucial and, even more so, for a child fighting a chronic disease.

When chronic illness leads to poor eating habits, a spiraling effect can develop. A poor diet results in nutritional deficits, such as iron deficiency, typified by fatigue and anemia (a low red blood cell count). As fatigue saps your child's energy further, she might opt instead to stay at home more often, snacking on junk food in front of the television.

Weight gain also is risky. Extra pounds place additional stress on your child's vulnerable joints. They discourage your child from staying active—activity she needs to keep joints flexible. Your child may feel worse about herself, affecting her ability to make friends. And so the cycle continues.

That being said, it's important to recognize that some children with arthritis face unique challenges in obtaining recommended nutrients. It may hurt your child to chew if arthritis has affected the temporomandibular joint (TMJ).

Some medications can suppress the appetite or cause stomach upset. Others may deplete specific nutrients. Calcium and vitamin D supplements, for example, may be recommended for children taking corticosteroids, which can cause brittle bones. Methotrexate can lower levels of folic acid and supplements may be recommended.

To address nutritional deficits, you may have to practice a little creativity. Worried that your child is getting too thin? Offer frequent, but healthy snacks between meals: applesauce, low-fat yogurt, whole grain crackers. When your child does eat a meal, keep the quantity reasonable, but take steps to bolster the calories and nutrients on her plate.

With the help of your child's doctor, you should schedule a meeting with a dietitian to develop some healthy and enticing food options. This will take some extra time, but it's important that your child does not cut nutritional corners, regardless of underlying weight issues. Your child's long-term health and short-term energy will reap the benefits.

A FEW EXERCISES TO BUILD CORE STRENGTH

Your child also can use exercises to improve and maintain good posture. The several below are designed to help by firming your child's abdominal muscles and strengthening the muscles of the back.

① Lie on the back with knees bent. Keep the back flat against the floor. Raise both bent knees toward the chest. Place hands behind thighs and pull toward the chest. Lower legs to the original position. While doing the exercise, be sure to pull in the belly button to work the deep abdominal muscles, thus protecting the lower back.

② Lying on the back with knees bent, place hands on abdomen. Tighten the stomach muscles and press the small of the back into the floor. Hold and release. Repeat at least several times, up to 10 times.

③ Lying on the stomach, lift the head and shoulders. Hold to the count of 5. Repeat at least several times, up to 10 times.

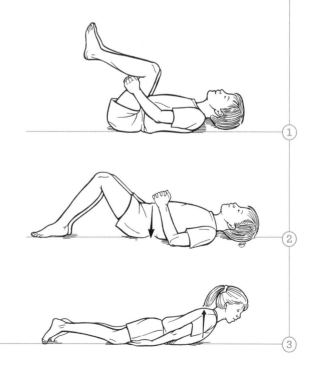

Wrestling with Fatigue

Fatigue can zap your child's well-being, making her daily tasks more difficult and eroding the overall quality of her day. In fact, fatigue can become so intertwined with your child's arthritis symptoms that it can become tricky to differentiate cause from effect. Fatigue can be a symptom of the disease process itself, causing your child to sleep more than usual. It can stem from inflammation, especially a flare. Your child also may experience fatigue from the physical and emotional energy required to combat painful inflammation.

VACATION: TAKING ARTHRITIS ON THE ROAD

Your child's symptoms have stabilized and that flare has receded in your rear-view mirror. Your family is eager to get away, to unwind and reconnect. With a little planning, you can start packing. Some items or logistics to place on your list:

DON'T OVERPACK: Use rolling luggage for your child and watch the weight.

MEDICATION SAVVY: Plan for the unexpected. Travel with more medication than you'll need. If possible, store meds in separate bags. If one bag is lost or misplaced, you'll still have a supply. Don't forget a cold pack for refrigerated medication and make sure your overnight accommodation has a refrigerator.

KEEP MOVING: To reduce joint stiffness, your child shouldn't skimp on stretching. Take rest stops on the freeway or walk the aisles on an airplane.

REMAIN ON TRACK: Unfortunately, your child can't take a break from exercises, medications and other arthritis interventions. And don't forget sunscreen, if lupus, dermatomyositis, another form of arthritis or the medicines she's taking makes her sun sensitive.

SCOUT ACCESSIBILITY: If your child uses a wheelchair, consider hiring a travel agent or a trip planner who specializes in accessible travel. When booking the room or trip yourself, get confirmation in writing. Ask to speak to someone at the hotel. The individual answering the toll-free number for the hotel chain may not have sufficient detail about specific rooms.

SCHEDULE RESTS: Don't forget naps, snack breaks and other types of down time. Otherwise, your child may push herself too much and pay dearly when she experiences pain or fatigue the next day. Sometimes, you'll need to split siblings between parents, so those without arthritis don't get too stir crazy while the other sibling takes a break.

SCRUTINIZE INSURANCE: To cover the unexpected, check out trip cancellation insurance. But scrutinize the fine print to make sure it covers pre-existing conditions, such as arthritis.

She also may literally be positioning her joints differently, to guard against pain, with fatigue as the result. Pain also may disrupt your child's sleep, as she shifts again and again on the mattress in search of relief. Or, your child may simply be fatigued because she has pushed herself too hard that day.

Sleep disruptions may be another cause of fatigue. Your child may sleep fine through most of the night before awakening an hour or two before the alarm. Your child may struggle to fall asleep or her night may be riddled with periodic awakenings. Even if your child appears to be sleeping, her sleep might be less restorative. At least some research indicates that children with juvenile arthritis are less likely to slip into slow-wave sleep, considered to be the deeper stages of the sleep cycle.

Besides the obvious immediate fallout—inattention at school and at home—fatigue can undercut your child's quality of life in other ways. Her lack of energy may sap her interest in exercise, social activities or recreation. She can become irritable, affecting relationships with friends and siblings. Your child may not feel like doing much of anything, further placing her long-term mobility and function at risk.

Another factor involved in fatigue is your child's activity level. Is she challenging herself enough—or too much? The right amount and level of exercise can boost your child's energy and alertness. But a child who pushes her body's limits to keep pace with friends risks exhaustion. The boomerang fatigue may not be worth it.

What should you do? First, make sure to raise the issue with your child's rheumatologist, so physical causes can be ruled out, such as iron deficiency anemia. Adjusting arthritis medication also could make a difference; with less pain, your child might get more restful sleep. You also might want to check whether her arthritis medication can be a potential insomnia trigger. Some drugs, including prednisone and hydroxychloroquine, can disturb sleep. One alternative may be to take them earlier in the day.

You also can help by reminding your child—likely repeatedly—about the importance of good bedtime habits. (Phone calls from friends, video games, a favorite television program—all can rob your child of rest.) Good sleep habits start with setting a consistent bedtime and sticking with it. Instead, establish a routine, including a warm bath or shower, along with the use of heating pads to warm joints. Big meals should be avoided right before bedtime; also limit your child's caffeine intake.

Try to discourage too much obsession with sleep, or the lack of it. Insomnia can become a self-fulfilling prophecy. When your child can't fall asleep after a short stretch, suggest that she switch on a light and read until her eyelids become droopy again.

A Parent's Role

In truth, some of the strategies for improving daily living may seem simple or obvious. But they can be forgotten or ignored amid the larger questions and potential complications of injections, therapy, peer relationships and other complex arthritis decisions. Try not to neglect taking some of these basic steps, like ensuring good nutrition and rest.

As a parent, you can play a large role in developing your child's mindset and ability to tackle daily tasks simply by emphasizing normalcy. You can positively influence how your child manages the rhythm of each day—from getting dressed to easily opening the front door. And that can influence the perception your child takes out into the world, of herself and her ability to handle the disease. ●

CHAPTER TWELVE

Shifting Into Third Gear: Movement and Recreation

Children, when they feel good, just want to move. Whether it's playing hide-and-seek or pushing pedals on a new bicycle, they are bodies in motion. Some parents can probably describe the exact moment when the medication kicked in and their child ran across the floor or started jumping on the bed or bounded down the stairs. Grating sounds, perhaps, for the parents of a healthy child. But music to the ears of parents who've witnessed arthritis constrict their child's movements and interest in exploring the wider world.

Still, there's that nagging worry, which you can't quite seem to shed. How can you encourage your child to remain physically active without placing vulnerable joints at risk? The good news is that exercise is not just possible, but vital, for your child to live her best possible life with arthritis.

Until relatively recently, clinicians often discouraged the pursuit of sports or intense recreation out of concern that the exertion could hamper joint stability or trigger a flare. But a growing body of evidence continues to reframe that perspective. It appears that the potential benefits of physical activity, tailored to your child's disease and symptoms, outweigh the risks of becoming sedentary. A diagnosis of arthritis doesn't—and shouldn't—mean a childhood spent on the sidelines. In fact, doing the right kind of exercise will make your child feel much better.

By staying active, your child can reap the cardiovascular and other stamina benefits, at the same time that she's strengthening her muscles and joints. One review of exercise training programs, published in 2003, found

TEACHING FLEXIBILITY
Jen Horonjeff's Story

When Jen Horonjeff was diagnosed with arthritis in the mid-1980s, the clinical advice dispensed about exercise was far more cautionary than it is today. Her parents were discouraged from enrolling her in soccer or gymnastics, for fear that kicking and other impact-type movements would damage her joints. But Jen's parents didn't want their daughter to be sedentary. So they signed her up for dance class—at age 2.

For Jen, that first class became the gateway into a lifelong passion for dance and movement. She went on to study jazz, modern and other types of dance at the University of California, Irvine, where she earned a double major in dance and biomedical engineering. These days, Jen supports herself by teaching pilates, a popular exercise technique based on strengthening and flexibility. Frequently, Jen's students have no idea about her mobility issues until the 24-year-old positions herself on the mat to demonstrate the modifications she's developed to protect her own wrists, hips and other joints.

"I do look like the pinnacle of health," she says. "It doesn't look like, on first glance, that any of my joints are deformed. But on second glance, you can see—I can show them to you."

Jen was initially diagnosed, at 13 months, with the pauciarticular form of the disease (now called oligoarthritis). But inflammation and stiffness have since spread to most of Jen's joints, including her knees, toes, ankles, jaw, fingers and hips. Besides coping with related eye inflammation—called uveitis—Jen also has been diagnosed with several other conditions, including ankylosing spondylitis, Sjögren's that children with arthritis who completed 30 minutes of aerobic exercise at least twice a week reported an improvement in joint swelling, pain and mobility. Those are just the physical payoffs. Encouraging your child to be more active also can boost her confidence and social involvement.

Not surprisingly, due to some of the muscular deficits that can occur

syndrome and fibromyalgia.

She's stubborn about permitting her symptoms to slow her down. After trying many medications through the years, she currently finds best relief with infliximab (*Remicade*). She's learned first-hand that exercise lubricates her stiff joints, even on those aching days when she's loathe to roll out of bed. Prior to her morning dance classes in college, she would throw a heat wrap in the microwave when she got up and then wrap it around her left ankle—frequently her stiffest joint. By the time she drove to class, she could move the joint more easily again.

Over time, though, Jen has learned some tough lessons about her limits, sometimes by hitting a brick wall. She's always disliked taking medicine, so during one stretch in college, deciding she felt great, she abruptly (and without telling her doctor) stopped her etanercept (*Enbrel*). The experiment

worked well for a couple months and then the painful backlash hit, with her joints becoming so stiff that her dancing suffered.

She also has developed a healthy respect for the value of rest and won't skimp on her requisite eight hours, even if that means cashing in at 9:30 p.m. Her energy constraints also played a role in her decision not to pursue medical school, with the prospect of 36-hour shifts in her future. "I had to be honest with myself," she says. "Could I have done it? Probably—if I wanted to kill myself getting there."

These days, as Jen contemplates graduate studies in kinesiology, she's helping others to build their body strength and flexibility, including some clients struggling with their own back, knee and other painful challenges. "I empathize with people," she says. "And then I help them to figure out the best way they can function."

> "I do look like the pinnacle of health ... it doesn't look like any of my joints are deformed."

with arthritis, your child may have some catching up to do. Studies have shown that children with arthritis—even those whose disease is controlled or in remission—have a lower capacity for sustained activity. Still, many kids with arthritis engage in sports and can even amaze those around them with their determination and ability.

Your child's doctor or therapist can help you create an exercise plan or choose activities suitable for your child. They'll be able to share important insights into her joint risks or vulnerabilities. Joints can be damaged, over time, when children are pushed—or push themselves—too hard for too long. As your child gravitates to specific recreational activities, you, your child and her doctor will have to weigh the risks and benefits of that particular sport or activity.

Keep in mind that opinions may vary. Exercise is a broad term, one that encompasses everything from the therapeutic exercises prescribed by an occupational or physical therapist to participation on a competitive team. Experts don't necessarily agree on the optimal activity, frequency and any one of a number of other decisions involved in designing a fitness program. At this point, studies looking at different exercise methods are small and limited in design, if they exist at all. So recommendations tend

THE HEAT/COLD DILEMMA

Your child hurts. Does she need an ice pack or a heating pad? The answer: It depends.

Cold treatments, such as an ice pack, are more likely to be advised within the first 24 hours after an injury. For example, your child's knee was banged up during field hockey and has become painfully swollen. Ice, which can ease inflammation and swelling, also may blunt the edge of a painful flare.

Heat is generally recommended for more chronic pain, such as the daily soreness of stiff joints. By warming the area, your child's muscles relax and blood circulation is stimulated. A warm bath in the morning might help loosen your child's joints before school. Similarly, an electric blanket on a low setting might help prevent morning stiffness.

When one approach doesn't provide relief for your child, though, you may want to try the other. Some safety precautions regardless of your child's preferred method:

- Don't apply the hot or cold treatments for more than 15 or 20 minutes unless otherwise instructed by a clinician. Allow the area to return to a normal temperature before reapplying the treatment.

- Place a towel between the ice or heat pack and your child's skin. Use the treatments only on dry, healthy skin.

- Don't allow your child to lie on top of an electric heating pad or blanket.

to be based on a clinician's personal exercise philosophy.

But doctors and therapists say they are more likely to encounter an inactive child than one who skates the joint-damaging edge. You can play a large role in attaining the necessary balance by encouraging your child to pursue a fitness passion and finding a way—working along with a doctor or therapist—to make that happen as safely as possible.

The Role of Therapeutic Exercise

The first step toward better fitness is likely the most boring one, from your child's perspective. By developing and following a routine of therapeutic exercise, your child can improve strength, joint flexibility and other skills key to better joint support.

Exercises fall into several categories. Range-of-motion (ROM) exercises help your child maintain or achieve the motion necessary to accomplish common movements. A neck exercise, for example, may improve your child's ability to glance at someone standing just behind her. Building muscle mass also is important; to that end, strengthening exercises may be recommended. Another key exercise component—aerobic exercise—helps build your child's stamina and cardiovascular fitness.

To be most effective, the exercises should be performed regularly, despite your child's possible lack of interest. An exercise plan is useless if not enacted and followed.

To encourage compliance, consider setting a regular time and location for your child's exercises. They should be performed on a firm but padded surface, such as a carpeted floor. A bed is too soft and doesn't provide sufficient support. If your child struggles to get on the floor, try placing an exercise mat on a low table like a coffee table. Also, consider doing the exercises with your child and getting her siblings to join in, too.

Although the exercises may make your child's muscles sore, they shouldn't cause any pain in the joint itself. The exercise should be halted if your child complains of joint pain. If your child's joint is actively inflamed—such as hot or swollen—only gentle range-of-motion exercises should be done. Your child also shouldn't place full weight on that joint. Most importantly, your child shouldn't launch into any therapeutic exercises before checking with her doctor or therapist to verify that the exercises are appropriately targeting, without overtaxing, her joints and limbs.

Some Range-of-Motion Exercises

The illustrations below demonstrate some range-of-motion exercises. Most work on a single joint, but a few work on several joints at the same time. These exercises shouldn't replace any regimen prescribed for your child. If you have any questions, be sure to consult one of your child's clinicians.

To make the best use of your child's time, consider selecting five to 10 exercises that will help those joints with the greatest mobility issues. If your child struggles to hold up her hand in class or reach for a book on a high shelf, then focus on exercises that work the shoulder. The goal is not necessarily to regain flexibility during active disease, but to guard against any further loss of motion.

Take note: Exercises should be performed slowly and smoothly without a jerking or a bouncing motion. It's particularly important to move slowly. When your child moves a joint, it should be to the point of discomfort, but not beyond. Ideally, the exercises below should be completed at least two to three times on each side of the body, and potentially up to 10 times.

NECK

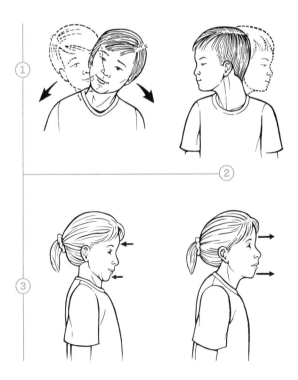

NECK

FIGURE 1: Tilt the head to each side, with the ear toward the shoulder. Don't lift the shoulder. Repeat several times, up to 10 times.

FIGURE 2: Turn the head toward one shoulder and then toward the other. Repeat several times, up to 10 times.

FIGURE 3: Start with the head facing forward, eyes straight ahead. Pull chin back like a turtle. If head is against a couch it feels like you are pushing backwards against the couch. Then push the chin and head forward like a turtle peeking out of its shell. Do not tilt the head up or down. Repeat several times slowly, up to 10 times.

PERSONAL STORY
....

SWIMMING THROUGH ARTHRITIS
Sarah Izzo's Story

Sarah Izzo spends almost as much time in the pool as she does on dry land.

The high school freshman hits the water by 4:45 p.m. every weekday afternoon, churning up laps for three hours before she heads for home. She also trains four hours on Saturdays and three hours on Sundays.

It was in the pool, several years before, that the first nagging pain hit her knee while practicing the breast stroke. Her parents first attributed the discomfort to growing pains, but it only worsened. Within a few months, Sarah got her diagnosis. "I remember when the doctor came in and said, 'You have arthritis,' the first thing that came to my mind was: 'Will I have to quit swimming?'" Sarah says.

Not a chance, as it turned out. For the first three years, a simple regimen of NSAIDs was sufficient to treat Sarah's disease, which has since been diagnosed as psoriatic arthritis. Until one day, Sarah climbed out of the pool crying, saying the pain was too fierce to swim on.

Her physician then switched the 12-year-old athlete to etanercept (*Enbrel*). From the start, Sarah was told she was mature enough to inject herself, says her mother, Debbie. The first time was hard on both mother and daughter.

Sarah, holding the needle, started to cry. "I'm very squeamish," her mother admits. Even so, she took a deep breath and turned to her daughter, asking: "Do you want to do it on me first?"

"Sarah said, 'I don't think so,'" her mother recalls. "She took the needle and—boom—injected herself."

In the nearly two years since, Sarah has learned to time her injections. When she has a swim meet, she does the twice-weekly injections the day before to maximize the medication's effect in her system.

Her arthritis, which primarily impacts her large joints, does place some constraints on her activities, including swimming. Her knees, ankles and, most recently, her hips are the joints most likely to throb, making the breast her most challenging stroke.

She has to limit impact athletics, stepping aside sometimes when basketball is played in gym class. She typically walks, instead of runs, when her swim team does laps on dry land.

Sarah's goal is to swim her way into a good college and further toward becoming a doctor. In Sarah's best stroke, the back stroke, she recently clocked 1:04 in the 100 yards, a time that she plans to put into her rear view mirror any day now.

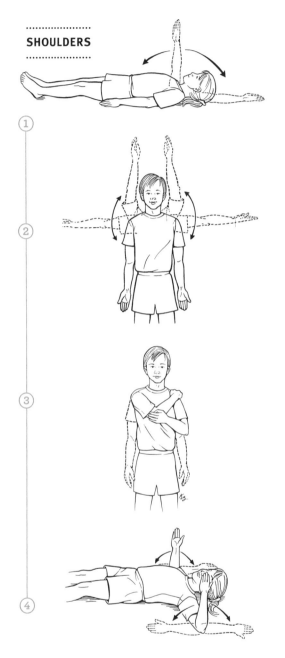

SHOULDERS

SHOULDERS

FIGURE 1: Lie on the floor with both arms at your sides. Raise one arm over the head, keeping the elbow straight, until the back of the hand reaches the floor. Return the arm slowly to the side. Repeat with the other arm. The exercise should be performed several times, alternating arms, and as many as 10 times.

FIGURE 2: Start with arms down at the sides with palms facing out. Raise the arms out to the sides and up until palms touch, keeping elbows straight. Hold briefly, then return arms to the side. If one or both arms are sore, it may be preferable to do this exercise one arm at a time. Repeat several times, up to 10 times.

FIGURE 3: An alternate position. Start with arm at side. Move hand to opposite shoulder and use opposite hand to stretch elbow across midline. Perform exercise with other shoulder. Repeat several times, up to 10 times.

FIGURE 4: Lying down, place the arms straight out from the shoulder, palms toward ceiling. Bend at the elbow with the fingers pointing toward the ceiling. Roll arms forward so the hands point straight down toward feet. Then roll arms backward so the hands point toward the head. Repeat several times, up to 10 times.

• **AN ALTERNATE POSITION:** Start with arms at sides with elbows bent to a right angle. Move hands and forearms across body, ending with hands on top of each other. Next move hands back to middle, then out to the sides and touch the floor. Keep elbows at a right angle through the exercise. Repeat several times, up to 10 times.

ELBOWS

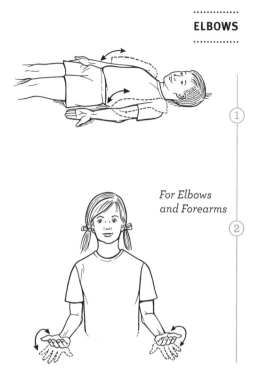

ELBOWS

For Elbows and Forearms

FIGURE 1: Lie on the floor with arms at sides, palms facing the ceiling. Bring hands to shoulders by bending elbows. Return hands to the floor by straightening elbows. Repeat several times, up to 10 times.

FIGURE 2: (For elbows and forearms) Bend elbows and hold them into the sides of the body, with forearms parallel to the floor and palms down. Slowly turn forearms so palms face the ceiling. Hold to the count of three and turn arms so palms face the floor again. Repeat several times, up to 10 times.

WRISTS

FIGURE 1: With the forearm resting firmly on a table top and the hand hanging over the edge of the table, bend the wrist up as far as possible. Hold. Repeat several times, up to 10 times.

FIGURE 2: Place the hand on a table or flat surface. Raise elbow toward ceiling until wrinkles appear at the wrist, without leaning on your wrist or otherwise placing body weight on that wrist. Repeat several times, up to 10 times.

FIGURE 3: Place the forearm of the wrist you are exercising flat on the table. Grasp that hand with the opposite hand. Put the palms together, with fingers around the opposite hand. (Make sure the pressure is on the palms and not the fingers.) Push the hand backward, stretching the wrist. Hold.

WRISTS

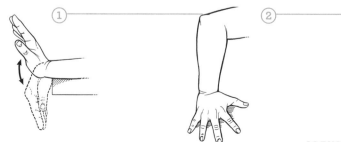

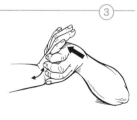

FINGERS

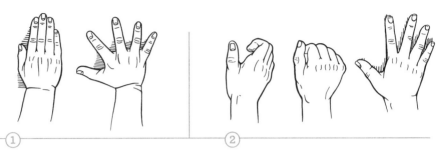

①   ②

FINGERS

FIGURE 1: Place hand and forearm on a table or flat surface with fingers together. Then separate the fingers as widely as possible and hold. Repeat several times, up to 10 times.

FIGURE 2: Curl the fingers tightly while keeping the knuckles straight, like a cat's claw. Complete the fist by bending the knuckles, then opening the hand wide. Repeat several times, up to 10 times.

HIPS

FIGURE 1: Lie flat on the back with legs straight, about six inches apart. Roll the legs in and out, keeping the knees straight. Repeat several times, up to 10 times.

FIGURE 2: Lie flat on the floor with the legs straight, about six inches apart. Slide one leg out to the side and return. Then perform the exercise with the other leg. Repeat several times, up to 10 times.

HIPS

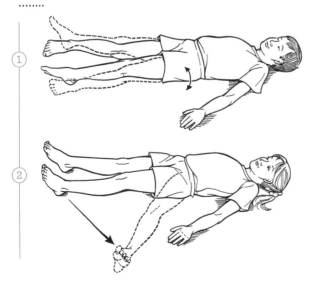

①   ②

FIGURE 3: While lying on the stomach, lift one leg. Try to keep the knee straight. Then lower the leg and repeat with the other leg. If it's too painful to lie on your stomach, you can stand and hold onto a counter or the back of chair, while lifting your leg behind you. If the exercise is done while standing, strive to maintain good posture. Repeat several times, up to 10 times.

FIGURE 4: Lying on a table with knees bent over the edge, bring one knee up to the chest. Place hands under knee on the thigh area. Pull in the belly button to work the deep abdominal muscles to stabilize the trunk. At the same time, keep the other thigh flat on the table. Hold for a count of 10. Lower the leg. Then perform the exercise with the opposite leg. Repeat several times, up to 10 times.

HIPS

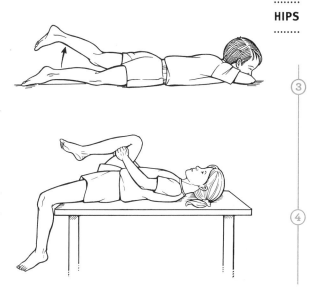

KNEES/LOWER LEGS

FIGURE 1: (For knee) Lying on the stomach, bend one knee, bringing the heel toward the buttocks. Then lower the leg and complete with the other knee. Repeat several times with each leg, up to 10 times.

FIGURE 2: (For lower leg) Stand an arm's length away from the wall, place both hands or forearms on the wall above the head. Extend one leg straight back, keeping the foot flat on the floor and the knee straight. The forward leg should be bent at the knee. To stretch the calf muscles, make sure the foot is pointed forward and not out to the side. Hold the stretch for 30 seconds. Repeat with each leg several times, up to 10 times.

KNEES/LOWER LEGS

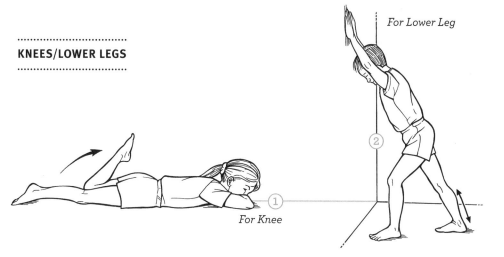

For Lower Leg

For Knee

ANKLES

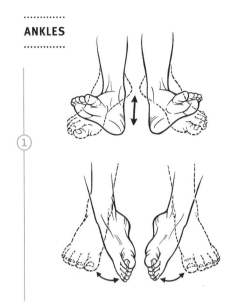

FIGURE 1: Sit on a chair with feet on the floor. Keeping the heels down, lift the toes up as high as possible. Then, keeping the front of the feet on the floor, lift the heels up as high as possible. Finally, turn the soles of both feet toward each other. Then turn them away from each other. Repeat several times, up to 10 times.

Getting in Motion

What if your child wants to step up her aerobic fitness, joining an organized sport or recreational activity like track or swimming? Should you grant your blessing? The answer, reached in consultation with your child's doctor, will depend in large part on your child's disease, as well as the jarring impact the activity can place on her most vulnerable joints. As your child's disease flares and ebbs over time, those recommendations may change.

In general, sports or aerobic exercises are believed to pose a lower risk if they are relatively low impact, involving large muscles used in rhythmic or repetitive ways. Some examples include swimming, walking in water or on land, dancing, bicycling and even running short distances. (After all, it's impossible to keep a small child from dashing across the backyard.) Doctors typically become more concerned when an activity puts stress on joints impacted by arthritis.

Depending on your child's vulnerable joints, those higher-impact activities might include gymnastics, volleyball, basketball, skipping rope or jumping on a trampoline. Running for long distances, such as for track or soccer, could be risky, particularly if your child has significant arthritis in the legs or feet. Doctors also pay attention to how much potential for bone-jarring collision a sport poses, such as with football or hockey.

None of these rules are absolute. If your child really wants to play a given sport or take a recreational class, you should raise the issue with your child's doctor or physical therapist. Sometimes with a little creativity, and perhaps some modifications, your child may pursue her passion. A physical therapist may suggest that your teenager with polyarthritis who wants to play volleyball do so but with some adjustments, including limits on practice sessions and more frequent breaks to rest the arms and wrists.

Remember, too, that an inflamed joint doesn't have to completely derail fitness. For example, say your child's knee becomes red and painful. In decades past, your child might have been advised to rest until that inflammation resolved. That approach not only fosters sedentary behavior, but also can put your child's nearby joints at risk of losing mobility and flexibility.

By working with your child's doctor or therapist, she can still enjoy some exercise. Water games and swimming are a great way to boost fitness with less risk to joints. Water can make a child feel buoyant and light when she feels clumsy or awkward on land. She also might be able to ride a bicycle, as long as the seat is adjusted to limit the degree to which the knee is bent while pedaling. Once the knee has recovered, your child can explore dance classes, soccer games or other fitness passions.

Signs of Strain

Children can push themselves—and thus their joints—too far. In reality, though, only a small percentage of children will risk damage to their joints. Typically those over-achievers are playing at the most competitive level, with one eye trained on the possibility of a college scholarship.

Children typically are smart about listening to their joints and making adjustments if the pain increases beyond their typical baseline. They may complain of pain when they move or touch a specific joint. You may notice swelling or she may limp at the end of practice, a red flag. They may, however, not tell you directly; a younger child may simply state that soccer "isn't fun any more."

So try not to cringe when your child plays hopscotch or leaps from puddle to puddle. She'll let you know when her joints need a break. You'll also be the first to hear when she wants to resume an activity. If you're still concerned, touch base with your child's doctor or therapist to get the green light. Then let your child go. ●

....

**GET MOVING:
THE YOUNG CHILD**
Even before your child is old enough to participate in organized recreation, she can enjoy informal games and activities with a hidden pay off—working her joints in the process.

Simon Says: This playground staple allows your child to move any and all joints. For example, you might say, "Simon says: Reach for the ceiling."

Tag or Red Light/Green Light: These games only require running for short distances. It makes it easy for your child to keep up or bow out when she feels tired.

Kicking the Ball: Roll a soft, light kickball toward your child and encourage her to kick it, which helps your child straighten out her knee.

Dancing to Music:
Young children love moving to the beat.

. . . .
Diagnosis and Family Adjustments

The diagnosis of a chronic disease like arthritis in a child can reverberate through the most resilient of families. It can hit you in ways that are both expected and not. The good news is that working through the challenges together can strengthen families over the long haul.

Along with the initial shock, anger, grief and other emotions, your family will have to adjust to the logistics of treating a complex and likely ongoing disease. Particularly in the early days, as your child's medication regimen is adjusted, your family's rhythm may be disrupted again and again—by lab tests, doctor's appointments, medication side effects and painful symptoms. Add to that mix the uncertainty of your child's future health. No doctor, no matter how talented, can predict the ultimate course of disease or how well your child will respond to medication.

These stresses, left to simmer, can expose fault lines in family relationships. They can turn up the heat on sibling interactions and rivalries. But it doesn't have to be that way, as long as you don't ignore or downplay your family's emotional reactions to your child's arthritis. By recognizing strains as they develop, your family can develop better communication and coping mechanisms. In the process, you also may learn how to reach out for

PERSONAL ESSAY

SHARING MY DIAGNOSIS
Jessica Stanley's Essay

Since I was diagnosed with mixed connective tissue disease (MCTD), I've had to answer a lot of questions from my friends and family. Some of their reactions annoyed me, others made me laugh. Almost every person said the same thing right off: "What the heck is that?"

I've lost track of how many times I've explained what an autoimmune disease is. At times, I wanted to put a sticker on my shirt that said, "I have MCTD" and give the Web site for the Arthritis Foundation so people could go look it up themselves. Some people thought the doctor had even made up the name to disguise the fact that he didn't know what was wrong with me. Others assumed that since the diagnosis wasn't something that was easily fixable, I needed to see a new doctor because this one didn't know what he was doing.

I get a lot of interesting looks. Elderly people look at me like they've never seen someone so young walking so badly. I've heard little children say, after I've passed them: "Daddy, what's wrong with that girl?" People I don't know stare at me in the school hallways as I try to make my way to class. When I first used the elevator at school, I heard a lot of comments, such as:

"You don't look sick!" or "You're too young to have arthritis!" I told them it would be nice if they could tell my joints that.

When a teacher mentioned that I should get a laptop instead of trying to write in class, someone asked why he couldn't have one. She said: "Jessica has arthritis. You have lazy. There is no assistance provided for that."

I'm on quite a concoction of medication. My chemistry teacher had fun figuring out what chemical compounds all the drugs contained. I told her the name of one, and she blurted out in the middle of class, "That is some serious sh—I mean, stuff!" Unfortunately, a side effect of the steroid I'm taking is that my face gets puffy. People who don't realize that's a medication side effect will feel the need to pinch my face and comment on my "chubby cheeks."

The most touching reaction came from my grandfather. One day, Granddaddy held my hand and said, "I am going to take this disease from you and give it to myself. It's not fair and I don't want you to have it anymore." And I know he really would.

—Jessica Stanley, age 16,
wrote this essay several months
after she was diagnosed with MCTD.
She lives near Richmond, Va.

help—to your church, a trusted friend or a therapist—and likely discover that you have more resources to tap than you had ever realized.

Processing the Diagnosis

Once your child is diagnosed, you may find yourself sifting through a variety of emotions, as you come to terms with the news and what it may mean.

You and your spouse may experience some degree of grief over the loss of a healthy child and your image, however realistic, of a seamless future. You may struggle with fear, both over the long-term uncertainties and over more immediate worries. Parents of a very young child may fear they won't understand what their pre-verbal child is trying to convey about her pain.

You also may wrestle with guilt, an emotion commonly expressed by parents. You may question your relative responsibility for your child's arthritis through genetics or actions during pregnancy or decisions after your child was born. Even though you know you are not to blame for your child's condition, that sense of guilt can be reignited repeatedly. You may feel guilty when your child is stuck for blood work, when she sobs over painful joints or, when—laceration to a parent's heart—you pin her down to inject the medication. Over time, that guilt likely won't completely fade. But hopefully you'll become more secure that your child's short-term discomfort has a long-term payoff in better relief of her chronic symptoms.

Talking to Your Child

Obviously, you are going to worry about your child's emotional well-being as well. How a child reacts to the diagnosis is highly individual, of course, but may be influenced by a number of factors, including age and an ability to understand the longer-term horizon.

A younger child may more easily adjust to the news of her diagnosis. An older child, say one approaching pre-adolescence and beyond, may have a more difficult time. By that age, she might better grasp the implications of a chronic illness and may fret over potential repercussions in the years ahead.

How should you discuss the diagnosis? Consistency is crucial. Before talking at length, sit down with your spouse and other key family members to discuss what you'll say and perhaps brainstorm some questions that might arise. You don't want different family members to send conflicting signals, without realizing it. As any parent can attest, however, a child can toss out a curveball question at any point. Even if you don't have a prepared answer, your previous "get ready" discussions will help give you an idea of what to say.

Adjust your explanations to not only what your child can intellectually understand, but what she appears prepared to handle emotionally. Listen for subtle clues. Is your child asking a lot of questions? If your child returns to one type of question, even in somewhat different ways, that preoccupation might signal that the explanation isn't clear or satisfying. Alternatively, does your child appear relieved that the conversation is wrapping up?

As you're talking, don't be untruthful or promise too much; that can erode trust on your child's behalf. Take care, however, to frame your answers in a positive light. For example, you shouldn't promise that the medication your child is taking will definitely work, but you can assure her that every effort will be made to locate the best medication. When you don't know the answer, admit it and say you'll make every effort to track it down—then do so.

This is really the first stage in an ongoing conversation, one that you'll revisit many times as your child passes through various stages enroute to adulthood. How you discuss your child's diagnosis will help frame her overall self-image and ability to handle the disease. Emphasize what she can do, rather than what she can't. (And, as new drugs are discovered, that list of limitations shortens.) You can live that attitude by treating your child with arthritis like any other family member, with roles and responsibilities. Such an even-handed approach eases tensions among siblings and builds your child's confidence when interacting with the world just beyond the front stoop.

Recognizing Feelings and Getting Support

To better work through emotions—yours and your child's—it's important to reach out for help when needed. Don't postpone that step for too long. Stifling feelings isn't healthy for anyone involved. You can't be expected to be happy all the time. Everyone has bad days or difficult times. Recognize them and give them their due, and let your child know it is OK to acknowledge these feelings, too.

Take advantage of support networks, including friends, family and your local church or community center. People want to help others. Call your local Arthritis Foundation office or request information from your child's doctor about any support groups or gatherings for parents or children with arthritis. Try to attend the national JA Conference to meet other families like yours. You and your child don't have to go it alone. Summer camps also provide a great outlet, allowing children with arthritis to share frustrations and build friendships in a setting where joint stiffness and injections are more the norm than the exception.

To release some feelings, your child might want to start a journal. Her outlet could be a blank spiral notebook or the computer screen. It can be used in myriad ways: to vent about pain, to discuss school conflicts, to write to an imaginary friend. By putting them on paper—or into bits and bytes—your child can begin the process of filtering out those draining emotions.

You may become concerned enough about how she's handling these life changes to seek out professional help. A younger child may develop a lack of appetite or become inactive for reasons that can't be ascribed to joint pain. She may opt to stay home, rather than to play outside with friends. An older child also may withdraw, but can act out in other ways by refusing medication or pushing joints beyond their safe limits. Grades may slip. Your adolescent may become even less talkative than usual.

Hone your parental instinct. Talk to your child's teachers and her doctors. But you know her best and can best determine if your child would benefit from seeing a professional.

Easing Family Stresses

The complexities of raising a child with a chronic disease can rewire the dynamics and interactions of the entire family—between spouses, between siblings, between parents and their children. For example, a child's medication regimen could interfere with the plans and routines of the whole family. Plans get cancelled, and soon the family's entire life revolves around the medication schedule of the child with arthritis. As a result, the rest of the family can start feeling resentful, like prisoners in their own home.

Family responsibilities may need to be rearranged. When one parent becomes overwhelmed by doctor's appointments, physical therapy and other commitments, the other parent may be required to assume more of the laundry and household responsibilities. The logistics associated with medication and other treatment issues also can weigh on both parents. Who is going to administer the shot tonight? Did you remember the other medication? Who will nag until the daily exercises are completed? Everyone in the household can pick up on that tension.

PARENTAL COPING STRATEGIES
Robin Soler's Essay

Arthritis is painful and frustrating. It also does not occur in a vacuum. We as parents have to deal with grief and guilt (lots of guilt), have to coordinate more than we thought possible and still have to deal with other major crises that come our way. And our children have to deal with these as well.

Life doesn't stop just because your child is hurting. You have to figure it out. I can't stop. I can't crumble for more than a few hours. When the kids get home, I am on my feet being a mom.

I think my initial ideas of coping involved what I crave most now—time alone to read, relax, cry, whatever. That is only a small part of coping and the part I am not so great at. But my educational training (as a developmental psychologist) and my own experiences with pain (I have

endometriosis and fibromyalgia) have taught me a great deal about ways to cope with all my family has experienced. There are a few things in particular that I believe have really helped.

SHARING: Sharing our stories and the stories of our children is critical. Some may call this venting. But venting is often associated with blowing off pent up anger at some immediate situation. Sharing is a calmer form of release.

I tell people about Isabela's arthritis all the time. I want them to know what she and other children experience. I want them to know that I am not distracted by fluff or tired because I was watching TV all night. I want them to know that I need help.

SOCIAL SUPPORT: The day I really learned to say "yes" was the day we first took Isabela to the emergency

Your healthy children likely have experienced their own conflicting feelings. They may feel guilty that they are healthy, overly responsible for their sibling with arthritis and resentful of the extra attention she reaps—all at the same time. After all, the child with arthritis gets to spend more exclusive time with parents, even if it's in the doctor's waiting room.

room to have her knee checked. My husband and then 6-year-old daughter, Elena, were there, too. Isabela had a very messy IV in her arm and there was blood in many places from other sloppy tests and fluid draining from her knee.

In the midst of all of this madness, Elena became very tense. My cell phone rang; a friend we hadn't heard from in months. I told her where we were. She asked if she could help. I said, "Yes, come get Elena." Within 30 minutes her husband had picked up Elena. That was the start of a long trail of "yeses" where I have built a mutual exchange network of sorts with people all around me.

HELPING: I find that helping my daughter helps me cope; I feel empowered in many ways. Clearly providing proper medical care is the first line. Getting her to the right doctors, getting her the right meds, getting those meds into her (this I sometimes forget to do and feel awful).

Putting a mattress on our living room floor for her to play on was a simple solution, but I felt such relief for just thinking of it. When Isabela had a physical therapist conduct home visits I asked the therapist to teach me all of the tricks she could in just three visits. (I was already overloaded with a gazillion co-pays.) Now I have all of these tricks—not just to relieve pain, but to get Isabela walking, stretching, jumping.

I also cope by helping at a broader level—participating in fundraisers and providing other families with information. By helping others, I have built a stronger and more reliable support network.

I've needed it. My husband suffered a heart attack five months after Isabela's diagnosis, followed by a major stroke last year. I use all of these techniques that I've picked up to get through each new challenge. Isabela and her sister also use some of them. I must say, I think they are working.

—Robin Soler, a behavioral scientist in Atlanta, has two children, ages 5 and 9. Her youngest, Isabela, was diagnosed with JIA at 12 months.

How can you help? Keep talking. Provide all your children plenty of opportunity to ask questions and express their worries. Look for ways to make them the focus of your time and attention. Spend an hour enjoying tea time with one child or set aside part of an afternoon for a bike ride with another. When you divvy up chores, or brainstorm about the next vacation, make sure all of your children are involved.

Also, talk with your spouse or other family members about the best way to tackle responsibilities of raising a child with arthritis. Negotiate who will handle what, and work out a give-and-take you can agree on. Write it out if necessary. Or if needed, bring in a trusted friend or relative to be an impartial person present during the discussion.

What Siblings Think

Your child's siblings will worry about arthritis and what it means—for the diagnosed child and the family. Listen carefully to their questions and concerns and prepare for them to shift as they move into preadolescence and beyond.

ELEMENTARY SCHOOL AND YOUNGER

Did I cause this? Many children think they caused arthritis by either hitting or kicking their sibling or wishing they'd go away. Reinforce that it is nobody's fault.

Can I get arthritis? Children this age may worry that the disease is contagious. The sibling may avoid contact with the diagnosed child, and friends may be reluctant to come over to play for fear of contracting arthritis. Be clear that arthritis is not catching and that it's OK for kids with arthritis to play with other kids.

MIDDLE AND HIGH SCHOOL

It embarrasses me when ... Kids this age hate to stand out. Having a sibling who is different may be embarrassing to the child who doesn't have arthritis. Over time, the sibling may instead focus on the strengths of his or her sibling with arthritis, rather than the differences.

You mean this may never go away? Children often do not fully understand the meaning of the world "chronic" until they reach their early teens. A sibling may think that, after a certain point, life will return to the way it was. It can be upsetting once they realize that it never will. Assure your child that children with arthritis live full, fulfilling lives. People with arthritis grow up to fall in love, marry, have children, travel, work, play sports and do almost anything anyone else can do.

Focus on YOU

As you race through each week, giving away pieces of yourself, don't forget to hold something back. It's important to horde a portion of your time and energy to refuel your marital connection and—lastly but most significantly—yourself.

Reconnecting with your spouse doesn't have to involve violins and an expensive dinner out. Schedule a night each week without the television blaring. Organize a babysitting exchange with friends who have kids. It only takes a couple of hours for you and your spouse to revisit a hobby, or you can develop a new passion—one that's for the two of you to enjoy.

Don't forget to find ways that you can retreat, whether it's for 30 minutes in a leisurely bath, an afternoon at the matinee or an hour at the gym.

Scheduling marital or personal time might feel almost stressful at first—like just one more item to weigh down your to-do list. It's OK. Give yourself permission. Tell your kids that you're scheduling "me time," or "Mom and Dad time." It's important for them to understand that parents have personal needs, too. After all, shelving that personal time for too long drains your emotional reserves, leaving you less equipped to handle whatever the next challenge is just around the corner. ●

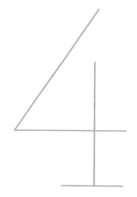

Ensuring a Bright Future

As your child grows up, external influences can multiply. We'll describe some of the stresses your child might encounter on the playground and in the classroom. We'll outline your child's educational rights, both in the lower grades and later into the college years. We'll be frank about the higher stakes of some risky behaviors, such as drinking alcohol, for those living with arthritis. You'll also receive financial guidance, from insurance issues to potential tax deductions. Finally, we'll provide a window into your child's future: career, parenthood and other transitioning issues.

. . . .

CHAPTER FOURTEEN

Growing Up With Arthritis

Growing up is never easy, or free from heartache. Like any parent, you'd prefer to shield your child from the various curveballs that life can throw her way. Some days the list of milestones, or potential obstacles, may loom large: making friends, handling sleepovers, changing schools, negotiating those first flirtations and taking risks.

A child with arthritis can handle all of that and more. Sore joints and surprise flares don't have to sideline her from the angst and excitement that's called growing up. But arthritis can sometimes complicate matters. Pain and fatigue may hamper your child's ability to cruise the shopping mall with friends or join a pick-up basketball game in the neighborhood.

As your child navigates adolescence, the complexities of arthritis and its treatment—from medication injections to therapeutic exercises—may present opportunities for rebellion. Peer pressure also may exert more influence, if your child is already struggling to fit in.

From an early age, you will have to lay the groundwork, helping your child to build a positive self-image and resiliency.

All children must learn to cope with peer pressure, self-esteem and other social stresses as they reach adolescence and young adulthood. Kids with

arthritis may face additional challenges, but they also have the same desire and potential to embrace life.

You'll always want to protect your child. What parent doesn't? Hopefully,
by teaching her to live with arthritis and not be defined by it, your child
will have more confidence as she ventures into the outside world. When
teasing or peer pressure takes its toll, she'll be able to rise above it. Painful
as the process may be, learning how to handle the inter-personal dynamics of making friends is part of growing up. Allowing your child to hide
behind arthritis won't serve her well over the long haul. Like all children,
she needs to build confidence to achieve the goals she sets for herself.

Building Friendships

Initially, your child's friends may not realize that she has arthritis. Earlier diagnosis and more effective medications, in many cases, have slowed
the emergence of the more visible signs of the disease. Because of this
your child may enjoy some latitude while building a circle of friends. Her
approach and willingness to talk about her arthritis also may vary significantly, depending upon her personality, age and maturity.

Younger children, those in preschool and elementary school, tend to be
more direct in discussing their arthritis. They may derive some pride in
their uniqueness. During those years, your child may allow you to speak
with her teacher about the disease and present some information to classmates. A brief presentation is a good way to answer questions and address any misconceptions upfront, such as fears that arthritis might be
contagious, or that children with arthritis can't play games or be hugged
without getting hurt.

With adolescence, your child, like many other teens, may close off some
of the communication channels you shared when she was younger. Your
teen may take pains not to stand out. She might choose to confine any
discussion about arthritis, and its related frustrations, to a close circle of
friends. Your child will make choices about who to tell again and again,
as she changes schools and meets new friends and, later, pursues romantic relationships.

Hiding her illness can be risky. Your child may push her body too far
rather than admit fatigue or joint pain. She may decide not to rest at the
edge of the dance floor or step aside when the gym class plays volleyball.

She may worry that otherwise she'll be left out, at a time when forming friendships and fitting in seems of utmost importance.

Teasing and Worse

Despite your best efforts, your child may become the target of taunting. Middle and high school students can latch on to any rationale—eye glasses, hair color or an odd-sounding name—as a reason to pick on a classmate. Arthritis may only provide another excuse to tease.

You can't necessarily stop the teasing—although you can intervene if the frequency or intensity crosses a line into bullying. But you can talk with your child about ways to deflect or discourage it.

Whenever possible, your child should strive not to become angry or teary. This will only feed the bully's desire for a reaction. Instead, encourage your child to ignore the ugly comments or use humor as a distraction. Also, your child should take advantage of safety in numbers. By forming a small core group of friends, she has defenders and will appear a less inviting target.

While common, teasing is far from harmless. It's considered outright bullying when teasing is done repeatedly and becomes aggressive. Nearly one in three students in 6th through 10th grades report being moderately or frequently involved in bullying, either as the instigator or the victim, according to an analysis involving nearly 16,000 students. Bullying was more common in sixth through eighth grades than the upper grades, and boys were more frequently involved than girls.

Other gender differences exist. Boys are prone to physical aggression. Girls rely more on words, spreading rumors or harassing via social exclusion. Over time, the stress can affect your child's health. One study found that headaches, sleeping problems and stomach pain, along with emotional difficulties—anxiety and depression—were more common among bullied children compared with those who were left alone.

It's difficult to stand back, but resist the urge to insert

....

SIGNS OF BULLYING

Federal officials provide plenty of information about bullying, including signs, causes and intervention at: **www.stopbullyingnow.hrsa. gov.** You may be the last to learn that your child is being bullied, as your child may not want you to get involved. Some signs to look for in your child:

- Returns home with torn or missing clothing or books.

- Has unexplained scratches or bruises.

- Appears to have few, if any, friends.

- Seems nervous about school or riding the school bus.

- Has lost interest in school work.

- Complains frequently about headaches or stomach aches.

PERSONAL STORY

ADOLESCENT ANGST
Wade Balmer's Story

Wade Balmer was nearing his teenage years when the contractures in several joints began to worsen. Unfortunately for Wade and his parents, his frustration increased as his condition deteriorated.

Since age 5, Wade had been coping with muscle weakness, red inflamed skin and other symptoms of juvenile dermatomyositis, an inflammatory disease primarily affecting the skin and muscle and sometimes joints. By age 13, Wade had developed a new symptom—calcium deposits that accumulated in his joints or appeared as nodules just under the skin's surface, causing pain when they were bumped or irritated.

Wade became fed up with everything: the doctor's appointments, the constant sunscreen and the nagging, flu-like, energy-sapping malaise. "I decided that the way I would take control is by refusing to do my exercises," says Wade, now age 29. "I would get into a fight with my parents every single night."

For nearly a year, he refused to do exercises at all, or only the barest minimum under duress. His parents tried pleading. They tried rewards. They tried reason, detailing the joint risks involved. And they were right, he says. "It's one of the largest regrets I have in my life."

It wasn't that those early teen years were uniformly miserable. Wade benefited from the companionship of a core group of friends. He flirted with girls. And his sense of humor helped him brush off, to some degree, teasing about his especially skinny physique that stemmed from a rare complication of his disease.

For years, Wade had secretly nurtured the hope that he'd reach a magical age—typically it was 18 or 20—and his disease would slide into remission. "As I started getting into my teens, that dream started crumbling."

His freshman year in high school proved to be the turning point. A calcium deposit had punctured his skin, leading to a dangerous staph infection. Wade spent two weeks in the hospital. His classmates rallied around, expressing their concern. Wade started talking more openly about his disease and its impact.

Nevertheless, the evidence of his adolescent rebellion remains engraved in his joints more than 15 years later. The contractures are most noticeable in his elbows. During that time, when he blew off his exercises, a crucial window closed, he says. "It's really hard to recover that flexibility if you don't intervene right away."

yourself into every challenge. See if your child can work out the situation. When you discuss what's going on with your child, listen more than talk. And don't minimize or downplay her feelings.

When should you intervene? The answer is highly individual and situational. Your child may suffer in silence, rather than risk getting you involved. She may fear that your efforts to alert a teacher or administrator will only aggravate her misery. But school officials may be clueless about the nature or the degree of the bullying. Alert them if you are aftraid for her safety. Sometimes prevention can be a solution.

Bullies can sense, and seize upon, a lack of confidence. To help buoy your child's self-worth, look for social situations and activities that will help her thrive and forge new bonds, such as Boy Scouts or Girl Scouts, summer camps and church youth groups. Encourage your child to get involved in after-school activities or programs in your community, where she can meet other children with similar interests. With a trusted friend or two, the wider world of childhood and adolescence can appear less threatening.

Meeting Other Kids With Arthritis

One of the best ways for your child to combat isolation is to meet other children with arthritis. When she does, her perception that she's the "only kid in the world" can melt away. Often, shared experiences or perspectives can make for fast friendships. And older kids or young adults with arthritis can impart wisdom about growing up that can only come from first-hand experience. Chances are that this kid-to-kid advice will sometimes ring more true than the wisdom that you or her doctors have tried to share with your child.

Unfortunately, for many families, it's rare to meet other children living with arthritis in their community. But there are other families like yours out there. The best way to get connected is through the Arthritis Foundation. Call 800-283-7800 or visit www.arthritis.org to find the office closest to you.

Local offices often hold events specifically for juvenile arthritis families. They can include a JA family fun day, social outings to catch a ball game or teen groups. Summer camps and conferences are also offered in some areas and sometimes there are scholarships available to defray costs.

HEAD TO CAMP: Juvenile arthritis camps—often held overnight—are developed specifically for kids with arthritis. At first, the possibility of your child staying a few nights or an entire week away from home may unnerve your child, and possibly yourself. However, take heart in knowing that these camps are designed to help build your child's independence and give her a fun experience that is adapted to her needs.

At arthritis camps, your child can make friends and learn new skills alongside others facing similar challenges. And activities are designed so kids don't feel left out. At camp, kids relate to each other's experiences and won't feel that they have to hide or downplay the fact that they have a chronic disease. The camaraderie is instantaneous and friendships can last for years. Some campers later become camp counselors as young adults.

Although the primary focus of camp is typically swimming, nature walking, arts and crafts, and other common camp activities, some education is included. So, along with picking up some new interests, your child may learn new skills for better managing her arthritis. There's also a medical staff person onsite, so when you drop your child off, you don't have to worry about her medications or a sudden flare—she'll be in good hands. Whether your child goes to camp only once or year after year, the connections she will make and the skills she'll learn can bolster her confidence in the years ahead.

CONNECT AT A CONFERENCE: While camps focus on the kids, conferences offer similar opportunities for meeting new friends and learning, but they are designed with the whole family in mind. At a conference—often held in a hotel or conference center—children are grouped with others their age and participate in activities while parents attend educational sessions. Parents can attend presentations given by leading experts that cover topics ranging from treatment and research advances to parenting and coping tips. Families share meals together, and at night, additional activities are often planned or families are free to explore the host city on their own.

The Arthritis Foundation holds a national Juvenile Arthritis Conference annually but its location changes from year to year. In some areas of the country, regional conferences also are available.

CRUISE THE INTERNET: Another natural meeting place is the Internet. Through online social networking sites and with appropriate parental supervision, people with similar backgrounds or interests can congregate virtually all while living hundreds of miles apart. The Arthritis Foundation offers discussion boards for parents on its Web site. There, parents can post questions and lend support to one another. Kids also can connect across the miles through the Arthritis Foundation's Pen Pal program. When your child signs up, she will be matched with another child with arthritis so they can stay in touch throughout the year. (*See the Appendix for more information.*)

The Internet also enables your child to keep up with friends she has met at arthritis events through various methods: e-mail, instant messaging and social networking sites. The convenience of cell phones also makes communication—through calls or text messages—much easier than before. So once your child does meet another child with arthritis, staying connected can be a breeze.

Risky Behaviors

Before you can believe it, your child will be hurtling toward those teenage years. Is she ready? Are you? Have you maintained open communication with your child? More specifically, have you attempted "the talk" that all parents dread?

Don't postpone discussing sex, drug use and other risky behaviors because your child seems shy or disinterested in the opposite sex. And don't assume that mobility difficulties or body-related insecurities will stymie experimentation. After a lifetime of rules and limits, your child might be more tempted to act out or push the boundaries to attempt to "fit in." And what's one more drug, your child might think, given the cocktail of medications she's already taking?

Research into substance abuse in teens with arthritis is limited, but one study from 1998, involving 52 teens, showed that nearly 31 percent had used alcohol. Other findings: 15.4 percent reported tobacco use and 13.4 percent reported using illegal substances, typically on an experimental basis. And since the teens self-reported their usage, the real numbers were likely higher.

There's also the potential for sexual activity. A 2002 study exploring sexuality and pregnancy in 246 adults who had been diagnosed with arthritis as children determined that nearly 38 percent had their first sexual experience by the age of 18; 7 percent were sexually active before the age of 16.

For an adolescent with arthritis, the risks of such experimentation are particularly worrisome. Some arthritis medications carry a risk of severe birth defects, if your child should become pregnant. (And despite myths to the contrary, the drugs don't prevent pregnancy.) Methotrexate, leflunomide (*Arava*) and thalidomide are among those medications most frequently cited for causing birth defects. The risk is so significant that your daughter will receive advice to stop taking the drugs for months, or take a special medicine to clear the medicine from her system, before trying to conceive later in life. It is very important to stress these risks and also to speak frankly about pregnancy prevention.

Meanwhile, alcohol and illegal drug use can potentially accelerate the side effects of the arthritis medication your child is already taking. Drinking in high school or college, for example, can be very harmful when your child takes methotrexate. The alcohol amplifes the strain that methotrexate places on the liver, boosting the risk of permanent liver damage. A teenager taking leflunomide runs a similar risk. For that reason, alcohol must be strictly avoided. Drinking also presents problems with other drugs. For example, drinking on top of nonsteriodal anti-inflammatory drugs can increase the stomach upset risk already associated with NSAIDs.

Unfortunately, cautionary messages don't always resonate with teenagers. In the 1998 study mentioned above, nearly 25 percent of those adolescents prescribed methotrexate also were consuming alcohol.

Don't assume your child's rheumatologist is raising these dicey issues. Various factors, including time constraints and awkwardness, can limit such conversations. One study, designed to assess the usefulness of a screening program at a large children's hospital, found that just 4 percent of patients were asked about alcohol use and just 12 percent about sexual activity prior to the program's implementation. It's important for you to raise these questions with your child and her doctor. Make sure that conversation gets started, even if it feels embarrassing or awkward to talk to your child about sex, drugs or drinking alcohol.

Facilitating Candid Conversations

Having "the talk" doesn't have to be one formal lecture, occuring at just the right time, when your child is the perfect age. To break the ice, watch for moments when you can react to something that's happened in the news or among your child's circle of friends.

As you talk, be honest and relatively brief. Monitor your child's reactions, watching for signs that she's engaged. When those eyes glaze over, that's a sure sign you've crossed the line from conversation to preaching. Books can help, to a point. It's important to remind your child of something she's likely not going to want to hear yet again—that she's different and behavior that's already risky for other teens may be especially so for her. Remember: most teens think they know it all, and that their parents just don't get it. Like any mom or dad, you'll have to persist to keep the communication lines open and let your child know that you're available to listen.

Make sure that you're candid and direct enough in your language that there's no lingering confusion. Your child must understand that she can become pregnant and that the risk of severe birth defects is very real. Your teenage boy with arthritis must also understand the risks of getting a girl pregnant.

You might be uncomfortable discussing drug or alcohol use, or sex, for fear that it conveys that you approve of your child participating. If that's the case, perhaps you can turn to a trusted friend, such as a godparent, to assume the responsibility of talking about these issues. Another option is to call the rheumatologist ahead of your child's next visit and request that the issue be posed.

Of course, your child will speak with the physician more openly if you're not standing nearby. The need for such conversations might also signal that your child is old enough to visit the doctor without a parental chaperone.

Preventing Isolation

Whatever your strategy, make sure your child has a safe outlet for communication. For many, the teenage years present a time to learn and stretch, to grow intellectually and developmentally. But it's also a potential emotional cauldron of insecurities, confusing feelings and peer pressures.

Your child can't escape being inherently "different" during a phase in life when the gold standard is to mirror her peers. It's important that you provide your child an emotional buffer, someone to whom she can download her fears and frustrations. Whether she confides in her godparent, a school counselor, psychologist or a friend, it can help her feel a little less like she's swimming upstream alone during this difficult phase of growing up. ●

....

CHAPTER FIFTEEN

Education: Advocating for Your Child

Some days your child may breeze into school, without joint pain or mobility issues breaking her stride. On others, she may struggle with the front steps, leaning heavily on the railing. Such is the unpredictable cycle of arthritis.

Don't let pride—yours or your child's—stop her from achieving success at school. Some aspects of school that most children take for granted can erode your child's energy and joints: hard plastic chairs, writing exams, long stretches sitting cross-legged on the floor. Modifications can be surprisingly low-key, yet provide significant relief. For example, to help your child flex stiffened joints, the teacher can request that she distribute papers or walk a note down to the front office.

Sometimes you can handle any concerns you might have informally by chatting with your child's teacher or principal. But don't dismiss setting up more formal and legally binding paperwork, such as a 504 Plan or an Individualized Education Plan (IEP). These plans are based on laws set up to protect a student's rights to certain accommodations at school.

At this point, such a step may appear unnecessary or potentially risky, labeling your child as different in the administration's eyes. But the educational rights and protections provided can offer some peace of mind, saving stress later on. All teachers may not be equally receptive to adjustments. Your child's schedule may change, requiring longer walks between classes. Or your child may awake with a flare the day before a standardized test, with no paperwork in place to provide for extra time for writing and other assistance she might need.

Back-to-School Basics

Before each new school year starts, and certainly when your child changes schools, you'll need to scope out potential headaches or hindrances so you can address them before they become problems. Some steps will be primarily logistical, such as setting up a medication system with the school nurse or administrator. Others will involve more subtle issues of communication and sensitivity, as you educate teachers about arthritis and what symptoms your child might encounter during the school year.

Your first step should be getting an advance look at your child's schedule for next year. Assess whether it's manageable, both in terms of the sequencing of classes and the layout of the school. Is your child slated to take physical education in the morning, when joints might be stiffer? How close are the classrooms to each other? How frequently will your child negotiate stairs? Is a nearby elevator available? To reduce uncertainty, visit the school with your child and do a trial run before the school year starts.

If your child must take medication during the day, you'll need to fill out the appropriate paperwork and likely speak with the school officials or school nurse as well. It's also a good idea to meet with your child's teacher. One of the challenges in educating others is the variable and sometimes hidden symptoms of arthritis. Pain and fatigue can sabotage your child's ability to concentrate and learn in school, in ways her teacher might miss.

To assist, provide each of your child's teachers with some literature about arthritis. (*For a sample letter to your child's teacher, see the Appendix.*) Request the Arthritis Foundation's brochure "When Your Student Has Arthritis." You also might fill out a checklist, with specific details of how arthritis impacts your child's day, from getting ready in the morning through school activities and homework. (*For a sample checklist, see the Appendix.*)

Another step to prepare your child: back-to-school shopping. By giving your child the best supports—from backpacks to shoes—you'll lighten the strain on joints and encourage her to practice good body-positioning habits.

Here's a useful guide as you embark on back-to-school shopping:

- **Backpacks:** Purchase a backpack that's supported in several places, including shoulder straps, a hip strap and possibly a chest strap. These straps distribute the weight along the length of your child's trunk. Then limit what you put inside. It's helpful if one set of textbooks can be kept at school and another remain at home. Another option is a rolling back pack, as long as your child can maneuver it while standing upright with very little effort. Look for one with shoulder straps, in case stairs become an issue.

- **Shoes:** Your child's shoes should be bought in advance so they can be broken in. They should have well-cushioned arch support and be sufficiently wide not to crowd the toes. Over-the-counter inserts may help provide better support. If your child wears a splint or an orthotic device, bring it along while shoe shopping.

- **Writing instruments:** To ease the strain on your child's fingers, look for pens or pencils with special wide grips or construct your own by wrapping foam—such as from a hair curler—around the writing instrument. Pens are easiest to use when they have a gel or felt tip, allowing the ink to flow more smoothly.

- **Workspace:** Check the desk or table your child uses at school to make sure its alignment doesn't unnecessarily wear on her joints. Your child should sit with her feet on the floor and hips at a 90-degree angle, with shoulders relaxed. Your child should not hunch over to accomplish her work.

Strategies to Plan Ahead

In a perfect world, a few conversations with your child's teachers and some savvy shopping would be sufficient to protect her interests. Still, the school setting or your child's disease might change, more quickly than you can anticipate.

At any point, you can line up the legal paperwork to formally detail the types of accommodations or services your child needs. One of the key legal protections available is the Individuals with Disabilities Education Act (IDEA). The federal law mandates that every child has a right to free and appropriate public education regardless of disability. One of the tools to accomplish that goal is an Individualized Education Plan (IEP), which must be developed for every child who qualifies for special education services. Once eligibility is determined, a child can access occupational therapy, physical therapy and other adaptive learning services.

In previous decades, when the mobility and other functional effects of arthritis were more pronounced, more children used IEP plans. In recent

---

Setting Up a 504 Plan
Jaime Moy's Essay

Prior to third grade, my son, Andy didn't have any formal educational accommodations in place. Until then, I merely chatted with the teacher before each school year. As my husband and I became more informed, though, we decided there were too many variables—perhaps one teacher might not understand his illness or the upper grade teachers might view some suggestions as "babying" him. We wanted to lay a foundation now to avoid any trouble later on.

The process took much longer than we expected—four months despite our constant involvement. But we learned some valuable lessons, through trial and error, along the way.

In July, I got the ball rolling by sending an e-mail to Andy's principal, asking to discuss a possible 504 plan before the Michigan standardized tests started in October. She replied that a meeting would be no problem; she'd get the proper paperwork together the first day of school. I relaxed. But I had already made mistake number one. Nowhere in the e-mail did I request a formal evaluation of Andy for 504 accommodations. That cost us valuable time later.

Once I received the evaluation forms, I forwarded them to Andy's pediatric rheumatologist and the social worker at the clinic. I soon returned the paperwork to the principal, along with a list of doctor-requested accommodations.

An informal meeting was scheduled for mid-September. Three people were present, including me. By the meeting's end, I had reluctantly agreed to let the school follow the doctor-requested accommodations informally until January. That was mistake number two; now the standardized tests were only a month away.

I expressed my concern a few days later to the principal and she years, children with arthritis have been more likely to use Section 504 of the Rehabilitation Act of 1973, which doesn't require your child to be enrolled in special education. Instead, it provides a broader definition of disability. Children fall under the law's umbrella if they have a physical or

immediately connected me with the school social worker. Once the social worker took over, she asked me to e-mail her a formal request to evaluate Andy for an IEP (Individualized Education Plan) or a 504 Plan. At this point, I also asked the Arthritis Foundation for help and they assisted with the wording. Via e-mails, the school and I communicated back and forth, but that led to mistake number three. Without face-to-face communication, we thought we weren't being taken seriously. On their side, the e-mails created tension, especially when we discussed timelines set forth by law.

Over the next few weeks, Andy was evaluated in several areas, including speech, writing, physical strength/agility and stamina. He also underwent psychological testing. The results only became available the night before we met with school officials to discuss eligibility. Thus mistake number four: I should have insisted on more time to review the evaluations, much of which was written in medical terms we didn't fully understand.

In the end, Andy didn't qualify for

an IEP, but did for a 504 plan. All of our requested accommodations were accepted and some added, including:

- **Pencil grippers for writing assignments when his hands don't hurt. A tape recorder, parent dictation or computer assistance when they do.**
- **Inside recess on very cold days.**
- **The option to use a pillow or a chair when the class meets on the carpet.**
- **Alternative gym activities, such as stretching or modifications, when his symptoms are active.**
- **An extra set of textbooks for home to decrease the weight carried to and from school.**
- **Additional time for written tests**
- **Less in-class work and homework when he's mastered a specific concept (example: 10 math problems instead of 50).**

As we wrapped up the meeting, thanking everyone, the speech therapist said, "And thank you for being such a great advocate for your son."

—*Jaime Moy lives outside Detroit, Mich. Her son, Andy, was diagnosed with juvenile psoriatic arthritis at age 5.*

mental impairment that substantially limits one or more major life activities, among other provisions. The law provides for accommodations.

As a result, students with some diagnoses, including epilepsy and attention deficit disorder, might fall under Section 504, but not qualify for special education services under the Individuals with Disabilities Education Act (IDEA). So might a child with arthritis, depending upon her physical disabilities and what type of services they need. If your child does qualify for a 504 plan, the plan that's drawn up should address obstacles specific to your child's symptoms. The plan, once developed, is a legally binding document that your child's teachers and other school staff must follow.

To the uninitiated, the various laws and plans designed to protect your child's educational rights may feel more like alphabet soup with all the acronyms and jargon. To help sift through the paperwork, you've got a number of advocacy and other resources you can tap, including the Arthritis Foundation or the U.S. Department of Education's Office for Civil Rights.

Setting up a plan can be lengthy, potentially consuming months, as the school district completes the requisite evaluations of your child, holds the related meetings and finally hammers out a plan. For that reason, advocates for children frequently recommend that parents complete the process even before your child needs accommodations so the paperwork is on file. In other words, the paperwork can be a form of insurance policy.

Before you launch the legal process, talk with your child about what you're doing and why. Explain that the goal is not to single her out, but to provide the support she might need, now or down the road. That conversation also provides you an opportunity to solicit your child's feedback on what aspects of school have been difficult and what changes might help. Children often don't like to feel different; you might question at some point whether you're overreacting. However, it's important to ensure that your child has access to every tool possible to achieve a successful school experience.

Making the Case

Since some children may qualify for assistance for both an IEP and Section 504 plan, one frequent recommendation is for your child to be evaluated for both types of eligibility at the same time. Typically, a school district will have designated one or more people to coordinate the 504 and the IEP process. Sometimes they can be the same individual.

As you pursue evaluation, keep notes of any conversations you have and place any requests in writing, beginning with the letter requesting that your child be evaluated. It's important to specify the special needs at issue and how they impact your child's ability to learn. One approach recommended by arthritis advocates is to use the following wording: "My child has a chronic health problem, arthritis, which limits strength, vitality and/or alertness and adversely affects my child's educational performance. I am requesting that he/she be evaluated for special services or accommodations that would assist my child in reaching his/her greatest potential in the educational process."

To determine eligibility, your child's school will request medical records from the treating physician and a series of evaluations, including cognitive and psychological testing. Once the evaluations are completed, a team will meet, including parents and the child's teacher, and perhaps a counselor or a physical education instructor.

The legal process includes built-in timelines to help ensure action. For example, once a parent submits a written request for evaluation, school officials have 30 school days to complete the evaluations and meet to discuss the need for an IEP. These and other time limits can be extended if both the parents and the school agree.

Despite the legal requirements, the response you receive from school officials can vary substantially. By sharing stories with other parents, you'll discover that there are not only differences between states and between school districts, but potentially between individual schools. The attitude of your child's principal, as well as how often a similar situation has been encountered, can influence how streamlined or difficult the process might be.

Negotiation Tactics

In some ways, the educational rights process might feel like an extended negotiation, with potential bumps and unexpected feedback along the way. School officials might argue that your child is "too smart" to require legal

---

ASSISTING YOUR CHILD: POTENTIAL ACCOMMODATIONS

With a 504 plan, your child may find that relatively minimal steps can ease the day's logistics, preserving her energy and academic concentration. Some possible accommodations include:

- Providing a padded chair to better protect joints.
- Shortening assignments to focus on key concepts.
- Altering a test format to minimize writing.
- Allowing the child to take notes on a computer or with a tape recorder.
- Providing a key to the elevator.
- Allowing extra time to walk between classes.

protections. They might discourage you from filing formal paperwork, providing verbal assurances that they can handle your child's arthritis needs.

As you embark upon the process, bring along the child's other parent or another advocate to join the meetings. They can take notes, ask questions and take the conversation down a notch if it threatens to become heated. Be direct about your child's rights without becoming aggressive or confrontational.

When the conversation seems to go astray, redirect it to your child's needs and how they can be solved. Find out if the school has encountered a similar situation; the staff members involved may be relatively new to the process. Ask open-ended questions. Inspire school officials to brainstorm with you about potential solutions. Play to their expertise as educators, and ask what they would recommend.

At the end of the meeting or the phone conversation, request a copy of the school's notes. If the school hasn't taken any notes, send your own letter or e-mail summarizing your understanding of what details were discussed. Another approach is to send a thank-you note, again laying out what was discussed. When it's necessary, reiterate the time tables set forth by law.

As with any negotiation, you may need to prioritize your desires for your child. Decide in advance which services or accommodations are most important to your child's education. Then prioritize other needs and requests accordingly.

Advocating for Your Child

Above all, don't take anything for granted. Depending upon the officials involved, resistance may not stem from a reluctance to work with you, but a lack of familiarity with the process. Do they cite a regulation as a potential hurdle? Request a copy of the paperwork and work from there. In the event that confusion deteriorates into stalling, or worse, reach out to a local advocacy group for suggestions. This is a great opportunity to network with other parents of children with arthritis. Learn how they achieved a resolution to similar challenges.

The bottom line: To be implemented, everyone on your child's 504 or IEP plan team must agree on the specifics. That includes you, the parent. When you're not satisfied with the results or the progress, you can work your way up the school administration ladder, right up to your designated school board member. Ultimately, if it's warranted (and hopefully it won't be), you can file a complaint with the state Office for Civil Rights.

Once your plan has been set up, stay on top of the situation to verify that it is implemented and appropriately updated, as needed, in the years ahead. With accommodations and services in place, your child's emotional and physical energy won't be sapped as much, so she has more ability to focus on the assignment at hand. ●

CHAPTER SIXTEEN
....

Finances:
Stresses and
Solutions

Medications used to treat arthritis have never been more powerful. They can now slow or even halt your child's symptoms in their tracks. But that effectiveness comes at a cost—in dollars, and time spent filling out seemingly endless insurance forms.

As newer medications are developed, their price tags can be breathtakingly high, from roughly $1,500 each month to more than $10,000 a month. Not everyone can count on health insurance to help cut the cost. By 2006, 43.6 million Americans—14.8 percent—were uninsured, including 6.8 million children under 18, according to data from the National Center for Health Statistics.

Those fortunate enough to hold an employer-provided insurance card have also been more likely to face restrictions in recent years, either in who's covered or how much the policy covers. Your insurance may not cover dependents, including children. It may exclude specific classes of medication. Or the policy your family relies upon may carry high deductibles that must be paid first before insurance picks up the bill for doctor's visits, medications and other treatment. According to 2007 data from Consumer Reports National Research Center, nearly one in four Americans face similar situations and are "underinsured," with significant gaps in coverage or high

THE INSURANCE GAP
Kerry Ludlam's Story

Kerry Ludlam, a journalism major, was two months out of college and still searching for a job. When a reporting position opened up at a suburban Atlanta weekly newspaper, she jumped at the opportunity.

She needed a paycheck, but it came at a substantial cost. The newspaper required employees to complete a six-month probationary period before they qualified for health insurance. "I had always been on my parent's insurance," Kerry says. "I wasn't thinking about how expensive it was going to be. I had always paid a co-pay [for medications or a doctor's visit] and that was it."

The lack of insurance would have been far more disastrous if Kerry took a biologic medication, which can cost at least $1,500 monthly, and potentially far more. But Kerry still paid about $200 each month for the hydroxychloroquine (*Plaquenil*) and other medications she took to treat her lupus.

Her boyfriend, who was already working, stepped in to help. Otherwise she couldn't have afforded the drugs on a salary that barely cleared $20,000 annually.

"Some men buy their girlfriends flowers and nice dinners," she jokes, wryly. "And he was buying me medication."

Kerry was lucky in several other ways. She didn't encounter an unexpected catastrophe, like a car wreck. Her lupus didn't land her in the hospital. But she hadn't anticipated the wear and tear on her system that came with working in the professional world. Gone was the college luxury of taking a mid-day nap or signing up for classes that started mid-morning or later.

When Kerry felt a flare developing, she would head straight home. She didn't take her chances or push the envelope. Rest was the medicine she could afford; she slept away many a weekend to stay as healthy as possible.

Eight months after Ludlam started her newspaper job, she jumped to a better paying public relations position with better benefits. The insurance consumed a larger chunk out of her paycheck, but most importantly, she qualified for coverage within 30 days.

> "Some men buy their girlfriends flowers and nice dinners... he was buying me medication."

deductibles. Even when you believe you've covered all your bases, a change in job or location can turn your insurance coverage upside down.

Sometimes insurance gaps or other pitfalls can't be avoided. But don't allow your frustrations to deteriorate into disorganization. Educating yourself on your options and keeping track of all of that paperwork and bills not only helps maximize your family's insurance coverage, but also may identify potential savings, including tax deductions.

Deciphering Your Policy

Despite shifts in the design of employer-provided plans, they still form the backbone of insurance coverage in the United States. But the types of coverage offered encompass a very broad spectrum, from those with low premiums and few restrictions to a more costly and less comprehensive approach. And the differences might not be obvious, at least on first reading. To prevent any surprises, you'll have to drill down into the fine print and compare policies when your employer offers more than one option.

To analyze a plan, make a list of what's covered and what isn't. To accomplish that, you may need to request a detailed summary of the plan, something more comprehensive than the booklet or marketing information handed out by the employer. When in doubt, ask your company's human resources contact for help.

Pay particular attention to laboratory work, physical therapy, surgery and any other types of medical services your child might require. Given the day-to-day fluctuations in arthritis symptoms, you'll never know when this information will become crucial. Are your child's medications on the approved list, typically called a formulary? If not, is there a mechanism to file a special request through your child's doctor to get them covered? For that matter, double check that your child's pediatric rheumatologist and other specialists are on the list of approved providers. Otherwise, you may pay significantly more for your child to see those clinicians.

Scrutinize the deductibles. That's the amount that you'll pay out of pocket before insurance picks up the tab. In many plans, well-child visits and preventative care do not fall under the deductible umbrella, but lab tests and X-rays do. Also, check out any total limits on coverage, such as annual limits per covered individual or for the family.

If you have the luxury of choosing between plans, grab a calculator and run the numbers for the worst-case scenario. Add up the premiums charged across the course of a year. Then calculate the cost of co-pays and deductibles based on the types of services your child might need if her arthritis flares. How do the plans shake out? You might find, depending upon the plan's structure, that paying higher premiums upfront can be cheaper over the course of the year, because your out-of-pocket costs will be reduced.

Once your family has coverage, do everything you can to keep it. Not only is an insurance gap risky in the short-term, it also can prevent your child from getting coverage when your family qualifies for insurance later on.

ADVOCACY: ADDING YOUR VOICE

Whether you realize it or not, you've become well-schooled in the art of advocacy by working the school system, the healthcare system and other arenas on your child's behalf. Consider applying those skills to the world of political action by asking legislators to implement positive changes for people living with arthritis.

The need for more arthritis-related federal help is great. Although arthritis remains one of the most common diagnoses, affecting 46 million adults—significantly more than the number diagnosed with diabetes (17.1 million), cancer (15.8 million) or breast cancer specifically (2.5 million)—arthritis-related research funding declined from $374 million to $339 million from fiscal years 2004 to 2007. Meanwhile diabetes, cancer and breast cancer research all received more funding than arthritis—$1.03 billion, $5.6 billion and $707 million, respectively.

But there is something you can do to help—become an advocate. Educate government officials by sharing the challenges your family faces living with arthritis. You can talk about the sky-high costs of medications and the stressful uncertainties. You can describe the long drives to take your child to the nearest pediatric rheumatologist.

From your perspective, these and other details may seem obvious, almost commonplace, but your representative or senator may not know much about juvenile arthritis. They may only have a sketchy awareness that children can develop this type of autoimmune disease. Follow your personal story with information on how they can help—usually by supporting legislation that makes funding arthritis research or related programs a priority.

Recent legislative initiatives supported by the Arthritis Foundation have promoted efforts to increase the number of pediatric rheumatologists, through incentives such as a loan repayment program. Another goal is to launch a national juvenile arthritis patient registry, which would collect data about the disease.

To get involved, you don't have to leave

By then, your child's arthritis will be considered a pre-existing condition. A federal law, the Health Insurance Portability and Accountability Act (HIPAA), generally requires insurers to cover a pre-existing condition if proof of continued coverage can be shown. The details are a little complex, and some exceptions apply. For more information, consult the Department of Labor (www.dol.gov). But in general, your child's arthritis should be covered as long as the gap between insurance plans doesn't extend longer than 62 days.

One way to continue coverage, after you leave or lose a job, is to take your home state or even your home. Contact your local Arthritis Foundation office and tell them you want to become an arthritis advocate. You also can sign up directly online at www.arthritis.org.

By taking that step, you'll be in the loop when Congress is poised to make decisions that involve arthritis funding and other initiatives. The Arthritis Foundation has at least 45,000 arthritis advocates. By providing your e-mail address, the Foundation can get in touch with you quickly, if your voice can make a difference for a specific piece of legislation. As an advocate, you might be asked to write a letter or e-mail your member of Congress or, if you prefer, to pick up the phone. You might be advocating for the legislator's support of a law or thanking him or her for an action that benefited children with arthritis.

For those who want to become even more involved, the Arthritis Foundation has recently added another advocacy program—Arthritis Ambassadors. The goal: to have one Ambassador for each of the nation's 435 congressional districts. As an Ambassador, you will be asked to commit typically at least two hours each month to reach out to your representatives on a regular basis and establish a working relationship. You may also be asked to help educate others in your community about arthritis advocacy priorities through tasks such as writing letters to the editor of your local newspaper.

Want to air your perspective in the nation's capital? Each year, the Foundation hosts an advocacy summit in which participants get a crash course in how Congress works, are brought up to speed about arthritis-related legislative priorities, and then, meet with members of Congress to share their stories. Your local Arthritis Foundation office will have more information on how you can participate, and some may have scholarship opportunities to make attending more affordable.

To learn more about the Arthritis Foundation's advocacy efforts and the most up-to-date legislative priorities, visit **www. arthritis.org.**

advantage of what's typically dubbed COBRA, for the federal Consolidated Omnibus Budget Reconciliation Act. Doing so could provide a critical bridge—at least 18 months and possibly longer—of coverage while you or your spouse searches for a new job with benefits. There's also a COBRA provision that allows young adults to continue coverage for a time, after they become too old to qualify for their parents' health insurance plan.

Again, there are exceptions; the right to coverage doesn't extend to people who worked for very small employers unless your state has additional protections. And the premiums will be pricey. You'll be asked to pick up the full cost, including what your employer paid, to be able to continue your coverage.

Shopping for Coverage

Families who don't have an employer-provided plan may still be able to get coverage for their children through the public system. The expansion of public programs, and most specifically the State Children's Health Insurance Program (SCHIP), has placed a notable dent in the number of children who lack insurance. In 2006, 9.3 percent of children were uninsured compared with 13.9 percent in 1997, according to data from the National Center for Health Statistics.

First created in 1997, SCHIP offers an insurance option for children who live in families who earn too much to qualify for traditional Medicaid but still below a set maximum income. The threshold on financial eligibility varies from state to state; so might the medical services that are covered. A child cannot be denied because of a pre-existing condition like arthritis.

Do you earn too much for your child to qualify financially for Medicaid or SCHIP? You might want to contact your county or state health department for further direction on your options. One possibility is your state's high-risk insurance pool, which is designed to provide an alternative for those—often with an ongoing or previous illness—having difficulty locating insurance elsewhere. For that reason, the premiums can be on the high side. Again, the specifics vary from state to state.

Paying for Meds

If insurance doesn't cover a biologic drug or another costly joint-preserving medication, the bill can quickly become overwhelming. One option is

SPEAKING UP
Nathan Everett's Story

The first time Nathan Everett ever boarded an airplane, he landed right in the heart of the nation's capital and political advocacy.

The sixth-grade Michigan student and his father had been asked to visit Washington, D.C., as part of the Arthritis Foundation's annual Advocacy and Kids' Summits. Every year, children with arthritis, along with their parents and other advocates, convene for several days. First, they receive training and education about arthritis-related initiatives, followed by meetings with members of Congress.

Nathan, an articulate 11-year-old, participated in a significant meeting with Rep. John Dingell, D-Mich. The long-time representative, elected from Nathan's congressional district, is chairman of a key subcommittee involved with arthritis legislation.

Nathan shared his story of being diagnosed at age 3, when an injured left ankle stubbornly refused to heal. He talked about how he was forced to stop wrestling after one knee developed arthritis. (He still plays football, baseball and soccer, among other sports.) "He refuses to define himself by this [arthritis]," says his father, John. "He refuses to go for pity. He has a lot of self-confidence, he's smart and he has a certain degree of charm to him."

After Nathan spoke, so did two sisters, both of whom have arthritis. During the course of the day, the Everetts also spoke with another member of Congress and at least four legislative aides.

The meetings left both Nathan and his father itching to do more. "It got my attention level to where I'm now motivated," John says. "Once I'm motivated, I tend to be kind of stubborn."

Prior to the trip, the Everetts had approached a local newspaper about Nathan's advocacy plans. A reporter wrote about Nathan's journey and his disease. After returning from Washington, D.C., John planned to contact the newspaper again to see if a reporter would delve into the legislative angle and write about the lack of movement on key arthritis initiatives.

Nathan, intrigued by the congressional pages and other activity on the House floor, now is more determined than ever to get his law degree. With that in hand, he plans to return one day to Washington, D.C.

> "He refuses to define himself by arthritis."

to contact the pharmaceutical company who makes the medication your child is prescribed to see if they have a patient assistance program for that drug. In the event that you qualify, after filling out some paperwork, you might obtain the medication for free or at a reduced rate.

Don't give up if your child doesn't qualify the first time you apply. The rules can frequently change and new programs can be launched for which your child might be eligible. Keep checking back to learn when you might be able to reapply. A good starting point for information about medication discounts is the Partnership for Prescription Assistance. It provides information on more than 180 pharmaceutical programs. (*For a listing of financial aid resources, see the Appendix.*)

You can take other steps to reduce medication costs, although the savings likely will not be as dramatic. Find out if your insurance plan has a mail-in pharmacy plan that provides you three-months' supply of medications at a reduced co-pay. You also can ask your child's doctor if a generic alternative is available. Although the latest drugs are available in brand name only, some of the older arthritis drugs, as well as those prescribed to treat stomach upset and other side effects, frequently have generic equivalents.

Don't be shy about telling your child's doctor if money is tight. In some instances, your doctor's first choice of medication may not have a generic option, but there may be another, cheaper drug that works nearly as well. Bring your insurance plan's formulary to the appointment so your child's doctor knows which medications are covered.

Maximize Tax Breaks

As the cost of your child's prescriptions and other medical services stack up, track all of those receipts. With some foresight and good record keeping, you may be able to get some tax breaks for all that money you're spending on medical care.

Take advantage of health-care flexible spending accounts if they are available through your job. They're becoming more and more common in workplaces. By setting up the account, you can request that a pre-set amount of money be deducted from each paycheck to deposit in that account. Money to cover health expenses will accrue over the course of the year automatically and be there for you to spend, while decreasing the amount of your income that's subject to federal income tax.

Another option is to open a health savings account, either through your employer or by establishing a separate investment account. Those accounts, which must be paired with a high-deductible insurance plan, allow you to accumulate money for medical expenses. Your contributions are tax deductible and any remaining funds at year's end can be rolled over to the next year or taken with you, in the event you change jobs. The money must be used for qualified medical expenses. Cosmetic surgery and most insurance premiums don't fall into that category. If you use the funds for a purpose that doesn't qualify, you'll pay income tax and an additional penalty.

Before establishing a health savings or a flexible spending account, it would be wise to consult with an accountant or financial advisor to gather more detailed information about contribution limits, eligible medical expenses and other issues. The rules can change year to year. Until recent years, for example, any money left in the flexible spending account at year's end was forfeited, i.e., "use it or lose it." Now there is a bit more flexibility, including the possibility of a one-time rollover from a flexible spending account to a health savings account.

Last of all, depending upon the size of your family's medical bills, you might qualify to deduct some expenses directly off your taxes.

To fall into this category, you'll have to amass significant medical expenses, as you can only deduct the amount that is more than 7.5 percent of your adjusted gross income. For an adjusted gross income of $50,000, for example, you would have to exceed $3,750 in medical expenses to write them off.

The good news is that you may qualify for a tax break even if your child's medical bills don't reach that level in a given year. You can claim medical expenses for the entire family, including all of your children. Plus, you have some degree of latitude in terms of what falls under the category of medical expenses. You'll have to check the specifics for your filing year by pulling down the appropriate Internal Revenue Service publication. In recent years, deductions haven't been limited to the more obvious—prescription medications, surgery, hospitalizations. You also can deduct numerous other items that you might not immediately consider: birth control pills, crutches, psychologist appointments, and lodging and travel related to out-of-town medical care.

Take note that some capital expenses also can qualify if you demonstrate that they assist your child with arthritis. Home improvements like bathroom modifications and ramps to the house are possible examples. As always, check with a tax professional first and document your purchases with receipts. Does your child's physician recommend a hot tub or water exercises? Request a prescription (if appropriate) or a letter specifying the arthritis-related purpose.

Wills and More

Paying medical bills may be one of your most pressing concerns today, but don't get too mired down in the here-and-now at the expense of preparing for future possibilities. Drafting a will, appointing a guardian for your child and purchasing life and other types of insurance all will help protect your family's health and well-being. By taking care of the legal complexities ahead of time, it will reduce the chance that you're child's arthritis treatment will be interrupted by paperwork, logistical or financial snags in a worst-case scenario.

The following are steps you might take to ensure your children are taken care of in the future:

APPOINT A GUARDIAN: It's difficult to contemplate, but you need to designate someone who will care for your children if both parents should die. Weigh all of the factors as you make that decision. Is this individual capable of raising your children? It's a huge responsibility under the simplest of circumstances. But when the emotional and financial challenges of arthritis are added to the mix, the duties of guardianship can become onerous. Before making a decision, talk with your guardian candidate to get that individual's input and hammer out any issues that might arise. That individual's financial stability is a crucial factor to consider if you're unable to set aside sufficient funds for your child's arthritis care.

GET ORGANIZED: To help your designated guardian, organize all of the requisite paperwork. Make sure the guardian has a detailed list not only of where the important documents are located, but any other aspects of your plan or decisions that you've made. Write out your rationale for some of your decisions, in guardianship and other matters. That preparation will be helpful in case your children raise questions later on.

PROTECT FINANCIAL ASSETS: Executing even a simple will can take months, so it's important to set up a mechanism so that crucial expenses, such as health insurance premiums, are not neglected. To that end, you should appoint a trustee. (To provide checks and balances, you might not want your guardian and trustee to be the same person.) Also, talk to an attorney about setting up a trust account for your children to cover immediate and pressing expenses while the will is in probate, or in the event it is contested.

REVISIT LIFE INSURANCE: You may already carry life insurance through your work, but is it enough? Talk with an insurance agent or financial planner about your need for additional coverage. They can run the numbers for you depending upon the specifics of your situation.

At the same time, it might be prudent to research other types of coverage. Disability insurance will help protect your family's home and other assets in case you're unable to work. Your risk might be greater than you'd anticipate. Studies show that a 20-year-old employee faces a three in 10 chance of becoming disabled for some period before retirement age, according to the Social Security Administration. Another item to check out: long-term care insurance. The coverage is designed to protect the family nest egg if you or your spouse develops health complications that require nursing home or other types of costly long-term care.

Practicing Perseverance

Like much with arthritis, the financial challenges of living with the disease can require patience and perseverance, more than you might be able to muster some days. You'll likely develop a detailed set of file folders and related notes. You'll learn more acronyms and jargon than you ever thought possible.

Keep in mind, you're not alone in facing these challenges. Alert your child's medical team if finances might threaten your child's care now or down the road. Publicly funded health programs, specifically SCHIP, offer more accommodating financial limits than were available more than 10 years ago. Local hospitals or medical centers may have charity programs and other resources your child's doctor can tap on your behalf. The last thing clinicians want to happen, after all, is to permit finances to place your child's joints at further risk. ●

CHAPTER SEVENTEEN
. . . .

Taking Flight: Your Child's Future

For years, you've been preoccupied with your child's next step—the first day of school, the first sleepover, the first dance and the first time she takes the steering wheel. And, then, suddenly it's no longer far off on the horizon; that exciting and uncertain chasm called life after high school.

Whether your child's chosen destination is a college or a career, she will soon be moving beyond your direct influence. That process has probably been unfolding for many years, even though you may not have been conscious of it.

When you've envisioned your child's transition to young adulthood, you might have considered the medical angles, such as locating a good adult rheumatologist or shielding your child from a gap in health insurance. But transitioning really is a multifaceted process. If successful, your child will gradually assume responsibility over her entire life, advocating for her educational rights to taking steps toward her chosen career.

To become fully independent, your child will have to separate from you both physically and emotionally as she embarks on relationships and moves and new jobs in the years ahead. For any child and parent, this period of transition is a challenging and sometimes emotional one, with steps forward and back. After years of battling a chronic illness together, it's a shift that might be even more difficult for you and your child to make.

Starting the Separation

Keep in mind that transitioning doesn't happen overnight, or even in a year or two. It's a process. The core of the transitioning process occurs as your child approaches her teenage years, but you should start setting the stage for independence years before, fostering self-reliance and confidence in your child, asking her to assume tasks and decisions appropriate to her age and maturity level.

By school age, your child should already be involved in taking her medicine and completing her exercises. She should be contributing to the household, handling chores alongside her siblings, albeit ones less likely to strain the joints. And by now, you've taught your child to recognize that

....

MAKING THE MEDICAL TRANSITION

When your child starts handling her own medical care, it can be tricky to know what she should be doing—and when. Although you should weigh your child's maturity and abilities when making those decisions, there are some rules of thumb.

YOUNGER KIDS (PRESCHOOL TO ELEMENTARY SCHOOL)

- Encourage your child to let you know how she is feeling.

- As appropriate, allow your child to be involved in treatment decisions.

- Teach your child the names of her medications, their dosages and when to take them.

- Have your child come to you when it's time to take medications. (For now, you should maintain control of the medicines and supervise the child when taking them.)

YOUNGER ADOLESCENTS (PRETEEN TO MID-TEENS)

- Continue to encourage your child to let you know how she's feeling.

- Begin to give your child more control over medication-taking. Have her take medications while you supervise, at first. Later, you may put your child in charge of taking her own medicine, but check in regularly to make sure she's complying. Encourage her to ask any questions.

- Allow your child to speak privately with the doctor if she wishes. Ask if she would like you to leave the room during the examination.

OLDER ADOLESCENTS (MID-TEEN THROUGH COLLEGE AGE)

- Have your child take responsibility for her medications.

- Ask your child to make calls to the doctor and schedule appointments, at first with your help.

- Work with your child to decide the qualities she would like in an adult rheumatologist. Help her contact your insurance company for a list of covered rheumatologists.

- Coordinate with your child's pediatric rheumatologist to transition to an adult rheumatologist.

some decisions, like jumping on the neighbor's trampoline, have joint consequences and to think those through ahead of time.

With that strong foundation of trust, your child will be better prepared to begin the more formal process of transitioning in her teen years, assuming more of her own medical and life decisions. One pediatric rheumatologist makes a point of flagging every medical chart once the child turns age 13 to start discussing the next stages.

For guidance on transitioning, you have plenty of help. Checklists and timelines, along with your child's doctor, can assist you in identifying which skills your child should have mastered by specific ages. The Healthy & Ready to Work National Resource Center (www.hrtw.org) is a good starting point, and makes checklists available. The American Academy of Pediatrics (www.aap.org) is another resource. For example, it's suggested that between ages 14 and 16, your child should start making her own doctor's appointments and requesting prescription refills. By age 17, she should understand her insurance coverage and how it works.

The beauty of starting the transition process early is that your child can take these steps with the support of a parental safety net. You can stand nearby while she calls in her refill or contacts the doctor's office to report a flare. Your child can spend short stretches in the doctor's office, speaking to the physician alone, gradually moving to longer stints until she eventually drives herself to the next appointment. As your child approaches high school graduation and starts looking at college or landing a full-time job, you can sit down together to research and discuss health insurance options.

To help facilitate the process, your child's medical team might ask some new questions, ones that extend far beyond physician checkups and medication adherence. They might delve into your child's hobbies and interests outside of school and get feedback about career aspirations, among other questions.

You and your child's doctor may need to push a bit to get your child's input. Typically adolescence is epitomized by teen efforts to self-identify and to hold parents at arm's length. But years of medical treatment and logistics may have made your relationship with your child, despite your best efforts, more interdependent in nature.

Your child may not be the only one reluctant to take the lead. Your child's rheumatologist also may have become too accustomed to your presence in the exam room and might need encouragement to meet with your child in private. Such one-on-one visits appear surprisingly limited. According to one 1998 study, nearly three-fourths of teens with arthritis reported never having spoken with their rheumatologist alone.

During this process, you also may need to take a hard look at your own emotional readiness. Don't hesitate to seek help, either from a support group or a professional, if you're struggling to give your child more

MAKING THE MOVE TO AN ADULT RHEUMATOLOGIST

At some point your child will need to make the move from pediatric to adult rheumatologist. It may happen when she graduates from high school or college. It may happen when she reaches a certain cut-off age, usually 18 or 21, established by the doctor. It may even happen sooner—when your teenager becomes uncomfortable sitting in a pediatric office with little kids. Regardless of when the transition occurs or is planned, here are some tips for making that shift a smooth and safe one.

PLAN AHEAD. You know the change is coming. Speak with your pediatric rheumatologist and take advantage of the time to plan. Chances are you'll have several rheumatologists in your area to choose from. What factors does your child consider most important—a young doctor? A male or female doctor? A doctor who is close to home? Ask your pediatric rheumatologist if he or she can recommend a doctor and help you schedule an appointment. Is this a good point in your child's disease process to change doctors?

CHECK WITH YOUR INSURANCE. If your child's pediatric rheumatologist recommends a doctor, ask your child to check if he or she is on your insurance plan. If not, suggest that your child share a list of covered rheumatologists with her pediatric rheumatologist. This step introduces your child to the reality that much of health care is ruled by insurance.

WAIT UNTIL THE DISEASE IS CONTROLLED. If your child is in the midst of a flare or beginning a new biologic, now is not the time to make the change. Experts recommend waiting until the disease is stable, particularly if your child has a disease such as lupus with risk of organ involvement.

DON'T BE AFRAID TO GO BACK. After your child's first appointment with the new rheumatologist, it's important to go back to the pediatric rheumatologist at least once to help ensure a smooth transition. Also, keep in touch with your child's former doctor to report on your child's progress.

latitude. It can be scary to allow your child to fail, particularly after years of protecting her from just that. But your child will be more reluctant to take the leap if she's sensing mixed signals from you. She might be more attuned to your feelings than you realize.

Selecting a College

College may be your child's first opportunity to leave the nest, to build a new life that's a drive or airplane flight away. It's a thrilling, but potentially nerve-wracking step for everyone involved. For children with arthritis, a little extra planning may be necessary, to help smooth the way.

If a four-year college seems daunting at this point, in terms of finances, academics or independent living, your child could start at a local community college, which typically offers lower tuition and a broader array of vocational programs. Once your child's interests have solidified, she may pick a trade or opt to complete her education at a four-year institution.

Depending upon the severity of your child's arthritis, the selection process might not rest solely on educational programs and resources. Your child also may be scrutinizing the physical logistics of the campus, along with the receptiveness of college officials to working with a student who has special needs.

Other logistics may come into play. Would your child prefer to be closer to home, in case her disease flares? Does the size of the college matter? A larger institution might offer more services, while a smaller school may provide a more flexible, nurturing environment. Of course, every stereotype has numerous exceptions. Also assess the geography of potential campuses. Are the buildings spread out? How difficult would it be to negotiate the hilly landscape? To answer these and other questions, your child should spend some time on campus, including a night in the dorms, if that can be arranged.

Rights at the College Level

In researching your child's next step, you might be surprised to learn that she can't necessarily count on the same educational rights that have protected her through elementary and high school. Most notably, the Individuals with Disabilities Education Act (IDEA) does not apply at the college level.

That doesn't mean your child doesn't have other legal protections. The federal Office for Civil Rights clearly stipulates that a college-level facility

FINDING A CAREER PASSION
Paul Felker's Story

In retrospect, Paul Felker can't quite believe it himself. Despite arthritis that dogs his joints—especially his hands and wrists—his career goal once was to become a music teacher or a concert pianist.

Initially, piano was supposed to be physical therapy to strengthen his joints and maintain flexibility for his polyarticular arthritis. But Paul quickly became hooked. He played and practiced through high school, entering college as a piano performance major.

Once there, the grueling collegiate practice schedule strained his joints. Toward the end of that first semester, Paul could only play 10 to 20 minutes, followed by 20 minutes with his hands immersed in hot running water before trying again. He practiced sometimes until 2 or 3 a.m. to avoid falling too far behind. But he never finished the semester. A "tremendous flare," as he describes it, landed him in the hospital.

That flare and subsequent recovery kept Paul out of school for nearly a year and forced him to reassess his future.

As he regrouped, Paul researched jobs, determined to make a wiser career choice. He discussed options with friends and family. He took aptitude tests. He wanted a career that he loved and could continue, no matter his mobility challenges.

It turns out that Paul didn't have to stray much further for his answer than the arthritis teen support group he helped facilitate at Children's Hospital of Philadelphia. One day a clinician there asked if he had ever considered social work.

At age 21, Paul returned to college with a major in social work. He went on to earn a master's degree, and is now partway through a PhD program. For the first 10 years, he worked in child protective services, reaching out to abused and neglected children. Most recently, his journey has returned him to the hospital corridors, working as a trauma grief counselor in the pediatric and neonatal intensive care units at Penn State Milton S. Hershey Medical Center in Hershey, Penn.

The therapy Paul has done in conjunction with his social work training has forced the 40-year-old, as he puts it, "to look at this disease that I have hated." He refuses to give arthritis any direct credit for his life choices, but recognizes that the disease has shaped him to some degree. "Through negotiating with arthritis, and the trials of it, it has changed who I am emotionally and spiritually and also my relationships with others."

must provide academic adjustments so someone with a disability can complete their academic work. But those protections generally aren't as broad as they are in the lower grades of education. And, unlike before, your child will be expected to advocate on her own behalf.

To negotiate the legal latticework, there are numerous resources available, including your local Arthritis Foundation office, the PACER Center (www.pacer.org), Wrightslaw.com and the U.S. Department of Education's Office for Civil Rights, which offers a helpful brochure to order or access online, called "Students with Disabilities Preparing for Postsecondary Education: Know Your Rights and Responsibilities."

Some key points to keep in mind, according to the Office for Civil Rights:

- Your child can't be denied access to her chosen school as long as she meets the admission requirements.
- Once admitted, your child doesn't have to tell college officials about her arthritis, unless she's requesting academic adjustments.
- To prove that your child has a disability, college officials will likely request documentation. An individualized education program (IEP) or Section 504 plan is generally not sufficient, although it might supplement other requested documents.
- Your child's college or university isn't required to provide a free appropriate public education, as public schools are in the lower grades. Instead the institution is required to provide appropriate academic adjustments as needed so your child can complete the required work. Your child also must have equal access to comparable housing that non-disabled students can live in, at the same cost.
- Examples of academic adjustments include priority registration, a reduction in course load, recording devices and the provision for note takers or extended time for testing. The school isn't required to lower academic requirements. For example, your child may be provided additional time for a test, but the test itself won't be modified.
- The college or university may not charge a student for providing academic adjustment. But college officials also don't have to take certain steps, such as supplying a personal assistant or a tutor. They also can argue that a suggested modification would significantly alter the educational program at issue or cause an undue financial or administrative burden.

This list is abbreviated and only contains baseline legal requirements. Your child's first-choice college may be willing to provide additional accommodations. To get a sense of the school's approach, carefully review literature provided by the institution about access and services for students with special needs. Each school also should have a designated person to handle any issues that might arise.

PERSONAL STORY

BECOMING A MOM
Jennifer Bolger's Story

Jennifer Bolger was the youngest attendee, by decades, at the educational class she was required to take prior to undergoing hip replacement surgery. And the 17-year-old likely asked the most startling question.

"I raised my hand," Jennifer recalls, "and said, 'I don't plan this anywhere in the near future, but what happens when I get pregnant?'" The two clinicians looked at each other and back at Jennifer, responding: "'We're not really sure.'"

That uncertainty about Jennifer's ability to deliver a baby vaginally would continue as she grew older, completed college and got married. She stopped her methotrexate, as recommended, six months before trying to conceive. Once she did become pregnant, she again asked physicians about her delivery options, given her hip replacement. "Nobody seemed definitive in their answers," she says.

Diagnosed with polyarticular arthritis at age 10, Jennifer has undergone extensive surgery over the years, some 15 procedures including the hip replacement. She spent a portion of her high school years in a wheelchair. In college, she withdrew from her Spanish and Italian classes after the pain and inflammation in her jaw affected her hearing and prevented her from opening her mouth more than a quarter of an inch.

But a year into her marriage, Jennifer's arthritis was stable on celecoxib (*Celebrex*) and methotrexate. She and her husband, Tim, decided to try for parenthood. Once she became pregnant, Jennifer stopped the celecoxib. For a few months, she took sulfasalazine (*Azulfidine*) to

Careers Choices and Considerations

Your child's chosen job or career might begin after high school, but it shouldn't be her first stint in the workforce. Holding down a part-time job or working as a volunteer, can benefit your child in a number of ways, as long as her academics or health don't suffer.

A job builds your child's confidence and provides a sneak peek into a

minimize joint pain and inflammation. By the second trimester, her arthritis symptoms had eased, as can occur with JRA during pregnancy, and she was off all medication.

It wasn't until the final month that the final burst of pregnancy-related weight gain proved to be too much for Jennifer's joints. She had difficulty walking or sitting. Her rheumatologist administered a couple of steroid injections. Still, concerned about inflammation in Jennifer's lower spine, the rheumatologist recommended a cesarean section at 38 weeks. Isabella (now known as "Bella") was born on a March morning; she weighed 7 pounds, 1 ounce.

Jennifer rebounded from the cesarean section. After a lifetime of pain and surgery, recovery was no big deal. She insisted on breast feeding until her joints couldn't wait any longer. After three months, Jennifer switched to formula and restarted her medication regimen.

In the months since Bella's arrival, Jennifer and Tim have developed a routine to bypass some joint-related frustrations. Before Tim leaves for work, he does some prep work, opening diaper packages and baby food jars and putting together some formula-filled bottles.

Less than a year after Bella's arrival, Jennifer is already contemplating a sibling for her blue-eyed daughter. But her rheumatologist has advised that she give her body a break for at least two years. If Jennifer does become a mother twice over, she plans to curtail work, another passion of hers. She currently directs a non-profit group that works with adults with disabilities in Jacksonville, Fla. For now, she's enjoying her first year with Bella.

> "By the second trimester, her symptoms had eased, as can occur with JIA during pregnancy."

number of careers. The work hours will keep your child engaged in the community and on the same track as her peers, adding to her resume in the process. Another bonus: She might pick up references useful for when she applies for college or a full-time job later on.

Selecting a job path is never easy, even without adding a chronic illness to the equation. You can help your child start thinking about options early. Pay attention not only to the academic strengths your child demonstrates, but also her other interests and personal goals. Talk to her honestly about any limitations in physical strength and stamina and how those might influence her career goals.

Notice if your child is drawn to certain hobbies or activities, like leading groups at camp or caring for animals. Pay attention to your child's personal style. Does she prefer to direct the crowd or is she more internally driven? Does she thrive under pressure or develop an upset stomach? Would you describe your child more as a big-picture type or does she immerse herself more in the details?

As your child gets older, encourage her to develop long-term goals. Would she prefer to have a job that helps others or make a product that someone can use? Does her dream life include running a business? How does family fit into her plans?

Your child should think big and not worry too much early on about how those interests will dovetail with her arthritis. Strive to be realistic, but not negative, about the job or career that catches her fancy. Your child's career focus might shift tomorrow—and numerous other times before job hunting becomes reality.

Plus, your child might be able to pursue another career in the same field, albeit not the one that first captured her interest. Depending upon the severity of her disease, working as a police officer on patrol might not be feasible over the long haul. But there are many other intriguing alternatives in the law enforcement field: the dispatcher who handles emergency calls, the lawyer who prosecutes felony cases or a forensic scientist who studies DNA and other evidence.

Future Paths: Parenthood

Since you're peering into the crystal ball of your child's future, you probably have contemplated another possibility: parenthood.

Arthritis may complicate the process of becoming a parent, particularly for girls. But pregnancy and parenthood are achievable goals if your child's disease is under control with minimal medication. Numerous adults, after living with arthritis for years, have gone on to raise families. And children who are growing up today are expected to find parenthood to be an easier path, thanks to earlier and more aggressive treatments that can minimize arthritis's overall toll on their bodies.

As with much in life, there are no guarantees. Your child's situation may vary from the norm, depending upon the severity of her disease, both now and in the long term. Before your child tries to conceive, she will need to consult with her rheumatologist, and likely an obstetrician, to discuss the logistics of getting pregnant and delivering a child. Men with arthritis will need feedback on the drugs they are taking.

Prior to attempting parenthood, your son or daughter also should evaluate—with some degree of honesty and foresight—their overall strength, energy and mobility. Can your child keep up with, and keep safe, an active toddler and young child? Is there a support system of friends and family nearby? And what's the willingness of your child's spouse to stay involved, given that support and assistance will be vital not just in the early days after the baby's arrival, but in the years ahead?

As you know firsthand, becoming a parent is about much more than the challenges and excitement of pregnancy and birth. It's a life-time commitment, one that's forged and strengthened through many years of challenges and learning and joy. ●

Conclusion

Living with a child who has arthritis, understanding her and helping her—is easier said (or written) than accomplished. Hopefully, you will feel a little less isolated, a little more self-assured now that you've read *Raising a Child With Arthritis, the* book on parenting when juvenile arthritis is part of your family's life. Simply by reading through these pages, you've already placed yourself ahead of the curve in managing the complexities of your child's disease.

We've provided you with a strong knowledge base. You know enough to question your child's doctor and health-care team members when something doesn't seem right. You have the skills to navigate insurance paperwork and school systems. You likely have a few tricks up your sleeve for those difficult days when your child is hurting and the medicine just won't go down.

We hope this book will serve as a touchstone, an ongoing resource that you can revisit again and again, when your child begins a new developmental phase or you crave some inspiration or reassurance from one of the personal stories or essays interspersed throughout the pages. And don't forget to turn to the back of the book, where a list of resources will introduce you to useful organizations and research literature.

As you well know, your education doesn't end here. You'll keep reading so you can make the best decisions for your child as she grows and matures, along with the science of treating arthritis. No doubt, there will be plenty of cutting-edge research to absorb.

While mysteries persist and not every disease—amid the dozens of rheumatic diagnoses—can be reduced to manageable levels, there is the promise of more innovative drugs in the pipeline. Advances in genetics will only further enable doctors to more rapidly match the best medication to your child's disease, without losing vital months to trial and error. There is so much hope in the field right now.

But the right prescription is just the beginning of joint-preserving success. Only you can ensure, on a daily basis, that your child takes all of the recommended drugs, completes those exercises and doesn't allow a diagnosis to prevent her from pursuing life's passions.

This generation of children, their joints buffered by the latest in pharmaceuticals, has reason to approach adulthood with far more optimism than any previously. As a parent, you can share in that optimism. Over time, your role will shift: from primary caregiver to supportive coach to, increasingly, a cheerleader from the sidelines. And, like any parent, you'll sometimes second-guess yourself or harbor fears that you're not doing everything you can to assist your child.

Try not to allow these parental worries to limit the scope of your child's world and what she attempts to accomplish. Be realistic, but not discouraging, in the face of your child's dreams. More than likely, she's surprised you before. As a parent, all you can do is raise your child, protect those joints through developmental years, nurture her strengths and aspirations and one day—sooner than you ever expected—take a deep breath and let her fly. ●

Appendix

Sample Letter to Teacher

Dear Teacher and School Nurse:

I am a student with arthritis and I would like you to know more about me. There are a lot of other kids like me (approximately 300,000 in the United States) but it is possible that because we are spread out all over the 50 states, you may never have had a child with arthritis in your class before.

There are some important things about me that I want to share with you. Sometimes I really hurt even though there isn't anything wrong with me that you can see. So if I am quiet, it doesn't mean that I'm not interested in school. Morning can be a problem because my joints can be stiff for the first few hours after I get up and sometimes by late afternoon I feel tired. A lot of the time I feel really good, but when my arthritis becomes active, I usually feel pretty uncomfortable. I hope this will explain why I have "up" days and "down" days.

I want to be in school whenever I can because I know that it is important for my education. I also want to be involved in as many activities and parts of school as I can. Sometimes it might be necessary to work out some special arrangements for me. I can't always take part in the regular playground or physical education programs. Sometimes I have a problem if the distance to the cafeteria or between classes is long or if I have to stand in long lines. I may need to leave school for a doctor or physical therapist appointment.

I hope you will have a meeting with me and my parents if you have any questions or concerns. My mom and dad will keep you informed if there are any major changes in my condition during the year that you should know about. The nurse at my doctor's office can also tell you more about my disease and answer questions for you.

I have the same needs for accomplishment and success as all kids, so I want you to have the same expectations for me that you do for all other children. I may take more time, but I can do the same things the other kids do if you will let me. If I can't finish my work on time, please let me take home my assignment to finish instead of excusing me on the grounds that I have arthritis.

Attached is a list of other challenges I may have and some ways to help me manage in school. I have checked some areas of concern that I currently have in school.

Thanks for letting me tell you a little about myself. If you have any other questions, please feel free to ask me or my parents.

Thank you,

Your Student

School Needs Checklist

You and your child can work together on this checklist or, depending on her age, she may be able to answer the questions herself. It can give her teacher a good idea of your child's strengths and weaknesses.

Have your child place an

A = always   S = sometimes   N = never   NA = does not apply to me

in the box next to each statement to describe herself.

GETTING READY FOR SCHOOL

☐ I can get out of bed without any help and without holding on to anything.

☐ It takes me less than 30 minutes to feel good after I get up in the morning.

☐ I must take a bath or shower to loosen up in the morning.

☐ I can go up and down the stairs when I first get out of bed.

☐ I can fully dress myself and put my shoes and socks on quickly in the morning.

☐ I have a lot of pain in the morning before I go to school to help me during the day.

☐ I need to bring splints, crutches, a cane or a wheelchair to school to help me during the day.

☐ I go to school later in the day than the other kids because of my arthritis.

☐ I take medication for my arthritis before I go to school.

GOING TO SCHOOL

☐ I can walk to school or the school bus stop without any difficulty or help.

☐ Waiting for the school bus is easy.

☐ I can get into the school bus without any difficulty.

☐ I need my parents to drive me to school or I take special transportation provided by the school.

ACTIVITIES AT SCHOOL

☐ I may need help dressing or undressing at school.

☐ I can go up and down the stairs quickly at school without any difficulty.

☐ I can use the elevator at school by myself with any difficulty.

☐ I need to get up and walk around in the classroom because of stiffness or pain.

☐ I can carry my own lunch tray.

☐ I can open my milk carton.

☐ I need to take my arthritis medication at school.

☐ I get embarrassed when I have to go to the school nurse.

☐ I can use the bathroom by myself at school without any difficulty.

☐ I find it difficult to write quickly.

☐ I need more time than the other kids to take exams or complete homework because of my arthritis.

☐ I find it hard to hold my pen or pencil.

☐ I find it hard to write on the chalkboard.

☐ I find it hard to use scissors to cut.

☐ It is hard to raise my hand in class because of my arthritis.

☐ I find coloring difficult.

☐ I find painting difficult.

☐ I get so tired at school, I want to rest.

☐ I'm afraid that some of the other kids will knock me over.

☐ I get frustrated because I can't always keep up with the other kids.

☐ I find it difficult relating to the other kids at school.

☐ I would like the other kids in my classroom to know I have arthritis as long as they don't treat me differently.

☐ I find it difficult putting on or taking off my gym clothes.

☐ I find it hard participating in regular gym activities.

☐ Playing outside in cold weather is a problem for me.

☐ Playing in the sun is a problem for me.

☐ I need to protect my hands form the cold.

☐ I get physical therapy at school.

☐ I get occupational therapy at school.

☐ I take a rest period at school.

☐ I get teased at school.

I find it difficult to:

☐ run

☐ jump

☐ hop

☐ skip

☐ play soccer

☐ play basketball

☐ play volleyball

☐ play contact sports

☐ other _____

AFTER-SCHOOL ACTIVITIES

☐ I need to take a nap or a rest period when I get home from school.

☐ I can finish all of my homework every night without difficulty.

☐ I cannot get through the school day and must go home early.

The type of arthritis I have is:

☐ juvenile idiopathic arthritis

☐ polyarthritis

☐ systemic juvenile arthritis

☐ dermatomyositis

☐ scleroderma (systemic sclerosis)

☐ hypermobility syndrome

☐ systemic lupus erythematosus (SLE, lupus)

☐ spondyloarthropathy

☐ psoriatic arthritis

☐ other _____

I developed arthritis in (year) _____, when I was _____ years old.

I currently have an IEP (Individualized Education Plan) ☐ Yes ☐ No

I missed _____ days of school during the school year _____ because of my arthritis.

Transitions: Changing Role for Youth

	Health & Wellness 101 The Basics	Yes I do this	I want to do this	I need to learn how	Someone else will have to do this — Who?
1	I understand my health-care needs and disability, and can explain my needs to others.				
2	I can explain to others how our family's customs and beliefs might affect health-care decisions and medical treatments.				
3	I carry my health insurance card everyday.				
4	I know my health and wellness baseline (pulse, respiration rate, elimination habits).				
5	I track my own appointments and prescription refills expiration dates.				
6	I call for my own doctor appointments.				
7	Before a doctor's appointment I prepare written questions to ask.				
8	I know I have an option see my doctor by myself.				
9	I call in my own prescriptions.				
10	I carry my important health information with me everyday (i.e.: medical summary, including medical diagnosis, list of medications, allergy info., doctor's numbers, drug store number, etc.).				
11	I have a part in filing my medical records and receipts at home.				
12	I pay my co-pays for medical visits.				
13	I co-sign the "permission for medical treatment" form (with or without signature stamp, or can direct others to do so).				
14	I know my symptoms that need quick medical attention.				
15	I know what to do in case I have have a medical emergency.				
16	I help monitor my medical equipment so it's in good working condition (daily and routine maintenance).				
17	My family and I have a plan so I can keep my health insurance after I turn 18.				

Transitions: Changing Role for Families

	Health & Wellness 101 The Basics	Yes my child/ youth can do this	I want my child/ youth to do this	I need my child/ youth to learn how	Someone else will have to do this for my child/ youth — Who?
1	My child/youth understands his/her health-care needs, and disability and can explain needs to others.				
2	My child/youth can explain to others how our family's customs and beliefs might affect health-care decisions and medical treatments.				
3	My child/youth carries his/her health insurance card with him/her.				
4	My child/youth knows his/her health and wellness baseline (pulse, respiration rate, elimination habits).				
5	My child/youth tracks appointments and prescription refills expiration dates.				
6	My child/youth calls to make his/her own doctor appointments.				
7	Before a doctor's appointment my child/youth prepares written questions to ask.				
8	My child/youth is prepared to see the doctor by himself/her self.				
9	My child/youth orders his/her own prescriptions.				
10	My child/youth carries his/her important health information everyday (i.e.: medical summary, including medical diagnosis, list of medications, allergy info., doctor's/drug store numbers, etc.).				
11	My child/youth helps file medical records and receipts at home.				
12	My child/youth pays co-pays for his/her medical visits.				
13	My child/youth co-signs the "permission for medical treatment form" (with or without signature stamp, or can direct others to do so).				
14	My child/youth knows his/her symptoms that need quick medical attention.				
15	My child/youth knows what to do if they have a medical emergency.				
16	My child/youth knows how to monitor medical equipment so it's in good working condition (daily and routine maintenance).				
17	My child/youth and I have discussed a plan to be able to continue health insurance after he/she turns 18.				

Reprinted with permission. Healthy and Ready to Work National Center, Maternal and Child Health Bureau, Health Resources and Services Administration

Glossary

Let this glossary serve as a reference for terms that are new to you while looking after your child's health.

Acute: Having a short and relatively severe course.

Anaphylaxis: Extreme sensitivity to certain medications or other substances, often resulting in shock and life-threatening respiratory distress; allergic shock.

Anemia: A condition in which the red blood cell count is too low.

Anesthesiologist: A medical doctor who uses drugs (anesthesia) to make certain a person is asleep and cannot feel pain during surgery.

Anesthetist: A nurse who administers anesthesia during surgery.

Ankylosing spondylitis: A type of arthritis involving inflammation in the spine that can cause the joints to fuse, or grow together. In children, the disease generally causes arthritis in the large joints of the lower extremities, such as the hips knees and ankles. Areas where the

tendons attach to bones, such as the heel bone, can become very tender as well.

Anterior: Situated in front of or in the forward part of an organ.

Antinuclear antibody (ANA) test: A blood test to determine whether certain antibodies that indicate an autoimmune illness are present. In children with some types of juvenile arthritis, the test can provide some indication of the long-term risk of developing eye inflammation, called uveitis.

Arthralgia: Pain in a joint.

Arthritis: Literally means joint inflammation (arth = joint, itis = inflammation). It generally means inflammation of a joint from any cause, such as infection, trauma or an autoimmune disorder. Term encompasses more than 100 diseases and conditions.

Arthroscopic surgery: Surgery done inside a joint, using a thin tube with a light at the end, which is inserted through a small incision. This type of surgery is best for minor repairs, such as removing torn or loose cartilage.

Autoimmune disorder: A malfunction of the body's immune system in which the body appears to attack and damage its own tissues. There are many types of autoimmune disorders or diseases, including arthritis and related conditions.

Biologics: These medications help control disease by changing the way the immune system works. They are developed using special technology from living cells, some that occur naturally and others that are created in a lab. They are most commonly used to treat rheumatoid arthritis and juvenile rheumatoid arthritis. They are also known as biologic response modifiers or biologic agents.

Chemistries: Your child may have other tests to check liver function, kidney function and other potential sources of their symptoms.

Chronic: Long-lasting or persistent.

Clinical trial: A study in which medications are tested in patients to measure their effectiveness and safety. This is one of the final steps in the federal Food and Drug Administration's process for approving drugs.

Clinician: General term for a doctor, nurse or other member of your child's health-care team that sees a patients in a clinic doctors office or hospital, as opposed to a health-care professional who primarily focuses on research.

CBC, or complete blood count: This test checks the red blood cells, white blood cells and platelets. Anemia, or a low red blood cell count, can occur with iron deficiency, or with chronic inflammation and can contribute to fatigue.

Corticosteroids: A group of powerful medications related to the natural hormones cortisone and hydrocortisone. These potent drugs quickly reduce pain and inflammation bur carry a risk of serious side effects when used in high doses. Sometimes referred to as steroids glucocorticoids, they are not the same as anabolic steroid drugs that some athletes abuse.

Cushing's syndrome: A possible side effect of taking corticosteroid medications; symptoms include weight gain, moonface, thin skin, muscle weakness and brittle bones.

DNA: Short for deoxyribonucleic acid, DNA is the building block of life. DNA holds the genetic plans for how your body grows, changes and ages. By examining it, scientist are also learning ways in which they can use DNA to predict the likelihood of you developing a disease and better ways to treat disease.

Dietitian: A specialist in nutrition

Discoid rash: A type rash that affects some people with lupus

Disease: An adverse change in health. Some physicians use this term only for conditions in which a structural or functional change in tissues or organs has been identified.

Disease-modifying antirheumatic drugs (DMARDs): Medications used to slow or perhaps halt the progression of disease. DMARDs are used primarily to treat rheumatoid arthritis and juvenile idiopathic arthritis, but may also be prescribed for other inflammatory diseases such as lupus, ankylosing spondylitis and Sjogren's syndrome.

Distal: Farthest from a particular point of reference.

Electromyogram (EMG): A test that measures electrical activity in the muscles. This procedure is used in the diagnosis of muscle and nerve disorders.

Erythema: Inflammatory redness of the skin.

Erythrocyte sedimentation rate (or sed rate): A blood test that measures how quickly red blood cells cling together, fall and settle toward the bottom of a glass tube. When inflammation responds to medication, the sed rate usually goes down.

ESR (erythrocyte sedimentation rate), or "sed rate": This test provides an indication of inflammation in the body, although by no means conclusive. Someone with a normal sed rate can still have arthritis. On the converse, someone with a high sed rate may not appear to be seriously ill.

Fibromyalgia: A noninflammatory rheumatic condition affecting the body's soft tissues. Characterized by muscle pain, fatigue and non-restorative sleep, fibromyalgia has no associated abnormal X-ray or laboratory findings. It is often associated with headaches and irritable bowel syndrome.

Flare: The term used to describe a period during which disease symptoms reappear or become worse.

Gastroenterologist: A physician who specializes in the diagnosis, treatment and prevention of diseases of the digestive tract.

Genetics: The study of inherited traits and how genes found in our DNA affect how we grow, develop and age. Discoveries made in the field of genetics have lead to some of the biggest advancements in treating arthritis.

HLA-B27 typing: A blood test to determine if the HLA-B27 gene is present. This gene is a genetic marker associated with an increased risk of developing arthritis that involves the spine, such as ankylosing spondylitis. Most children with this gene are healthy, but they are more likely than others to develop this arthritis. Your child can test negative and still have this arthritis diagnosed.

Immune response: Activation of the body's immune system to defend itself against foreign substances, or antigens.

Immune system: Your body's complex biochemical system for defending itself against bacteria, viruses, wounds and other injuries. Among the many components of the system are a variety of cells (such as T cells), organs (such as the lymph glands) and chemicals (such as histamine and prostaglandins).

Inflammation: A reaction to injury or infection resulting in redness, pain, swelling and stiffness in the affected areas.

Internist: A physician who specializes in internal medicine: Sometimes called a primary care physician.

Iridocyclitis (iritis, uveitis): A serious eye inflammation that is difficult to detect. Permanent eye damage can be avoided by having regular eye exams by an ophthalmologist. The term an eye doctor uses to refer to the condition depends on which part of the eye is affected.

Joint replacement surgery: Surgery in which diseased joints are replaced with man-made joints. This procedure is used mainly in older children and adults whose growth is complete and whose joints are badly damaged by arthritis.

Dermatomyositis: An inflammatory disease that causes a skin rash and muscle weakness. Approximately 20 percent of children with JDMS have arthritis. JDMS is more common in girls and occurs most often in children between the ages of 5 and 14.

Juvenile: Often used before another term to indicate it affects children. For example, juvenile lupus, juvenile diabetes.

Juvenile arthritis (JA): A general term used to describe the more than 100 rheumatic diseases and conditions that can affect children. Think of it as the term to describe arthritis in kids. JA can cover many diseases including lupus, fibromyalgia and psoriatic arthritis. Not to be confused with JIA (see below).

Juvenile idiopathic arthritis (JIA): The preferred term used by researchers, and increasingly doctors, to describe chronic, inflammatory autoimmune disease in which the body's protective immune system attacks its own tissues, particularly the joints, causing pain, swelling and deformity. JIA is the most common type of arthritis that affects children, and there are many forms of the condition. The three most common categories are:

oligoarticular: Formerly known as pauciarticular, at diagnosis it affects four or fewer joints, usually the large joints such as knees, ankles or elbows. Approximately 40 percent of children with JIA have this form

polyarthritis: Affects five or more joints, at diagnosis, usually affecting the same joint on both sides of the body. Affects girls more often than boys. Approximately 25 percent of children with JIA have this form.

systemic: Affects both the joints and internal organs, and can begin with a very high fever, rash, swollen joints and pain. Other forms include Enthesitis-related and juvenile psoriatic arthritis, among others.

Juvenile rheumatoid arthritis (JRA): An older term used to describe chronic, inflammatory autoimmune disease in which the body's protective immune system attacks its own tissues, particularly the joints, causing pain, swelling and deformity. For more information see JIA (*above*).

Lyme disease: A inflammatory disorder characterized by a skin rash, followed in weeks or months by symptoms in the central nervous system, cardiovascular system and joints. It is caused by the bite of an infected deer tick. The disease is named after the Connecticut town where it was first discovered. It is now found across the United States.

Malar rash: A rash appearing on the cheeks: also called a "butterfly rash" because of its shape. It is sometimes a symptom of systemic lupus erythematosus or lupus.

Medical journal: A publication either on print or online where research results are published in the form of articles.

Mixed connective tissue disease (MCTD): A syndrome with a mixture of symptoms of systemic lupus erythematosus, polmyositis and other rheumatic diseases. MCTD is very rare in children.

Myofascial pain syndrome: A neuromuscular condition in which the tissue surrounding muscles tightens and loses elasticity, causing pain and loss of motion.

Myopathy: Any disease of a muscle.

Myositis: Inflammation of a muscle. This term is used to describe several different illnesses, including polymyositis, dermatomyositis and inclusion body myositis. These conditions involve chronic muscle inflammation, leading to muscle weakness.

Nephrologist: A physician who specializes in the diagnosis, treatment and prevention of kidney problem.

Neurologist: A physician who specialized in the diagnosis, treatment and prevention of nervous system disorders.

Non-acetylated salicylates: Medications that are similar to aspirin but have been chemically modified to be easier on the stomach and kidneys and are taken less frequently than regular aspirin.

Nonsteroidal anti-inflammatory drugs (NASIDs): Medications that relieve pain, fever and inflammation. These are often prescribed to treat arthritis inflammation and pain.

Occupational therapist: A health professional who teaches patients ways to reduce strain on joints while performing everyday activities. Occupational therapists also fit patients with splints and other devices to help reduce strain on joints.

Oncogenesis: Development of a new abnormal growth or tumor.

Ophthalmologist: A physician who specialized in the diagnosis and medical and surgical treatment of diseases and defects of the eye.

Orthopaedic surgeon: A surgeon who specializes in surgery of the musculoskeletal system, its joints and related structures.

Osteopenia: The term for bone mass that is lower than usual but does not require treatment with medication unless there are special risk factors.

Osteoporosis: A condition resulting in the thinning of bones and an increased susceptibility to fractures. Unfortunately, corticosteroids, sometimes used in treating children with arthritis, can increase the risk of osteoporosis when used in children in high doses for extended periods of time.

Pediatric rheumatologist: A physician who has special training in the care of children and adolescents with arthritis and related conditions.

Pediatrician: A physician who has special training in the diagnosis, treatment and prevention of childhood and adolescent illnesses.

Peer review article: This refers to a type of research article that has been through the peer review process of having other doctors or health-care providers reading the article and helping approve it for publication before it is printed in a medical journal. Because of this extra layer of review these articles are viewed as being a reliable source for research information.

Photosensitivity: An abnormally heightened reaction to sunlight.

Physiatrist: A physician who specializes in the field of physical medicine and rehabilitation.

Physical therapist: A licensed health professional who is a specialist in the use of exercises to treat physical conditions.

Podiatrist: A health professional who specializes in the study and care of the foot, including medical and surgical treatment.

Polymyositis/dermatomyositis: Related rheumatic diseases that cause weakness and inflammation of muscles.

Primary Care Physician: A physician who specializes in internal medicine: Sometimes called an internist.

Proximal: Nearest; closest to any point of reference. The opposite of distal.

Psoriasis: A chronic skin disease characterized by scaly, reddish patches. Psoriasis also causes lifting of the nails and pitting, a condition in which the nails become marked with several small depressions.

Psoriatic arthritis: A type of arthritis that may occur with the skin condition psoriasis. Skin symptoms in children include nail pitting or ridging, and atypical rash behind the ears, on the eyelids, elbows, knees and at the scalp line or the umbilicus. Arthritis may involve both large and small joints, usually asymmetrically: The spine may also be involved.

Psychiatrist: A medical doctor who specializes in the study, treatment and prevention of mental disorders. A psychiatrist may provide counseling and prescribe medicines and other therapies.

Psychologist: A mental health-care professional who has received training in counseling and administering therapy. However, because they are not medical doctors, most may not prescribe medications.

Pulmonologist: A physician who specializes in the diagnosis, treatment and prevention of lung disorders.

Raynaud's phenomenon: An extreme sensitivity to cold that causes narrowing of the blood vessels in the fingers along with a sensation of tingling or numbness, and color changes to the skin.

Reactive arthritis: A form of arthritis that develops as a reaction to certain types of infections.

Remission: A period of time when the symptoms of a disease or condition improve or even disappear altogether.

Review article: Review articles attempt to gather all the research data on one topic that can be found in numerous studies and summarize it. They are good for getting a broad understanding of a topic.

Reye's syndrome: A rare, serious condition that sometimes occurs in children who have the chicken pox or flu and are taking aspirin. Symptoms include frequent vomiting, very painful headaches, unusual behavior, extreme tiredness and disorientation.

Rheumatic diseases: A general term referring to conditions characterized by pain and stiffness of the joints or muscles. The term is often used interchangeably with "arthritis", but not all rheumatic disease affects the joints or involves inflammation.

Rheumatoid factor (RF): An antibody that appears in unusually high amounts in the blood of some people with rheumatoid arthritis.

Rheumatoid factor (RF) test: A test to detect rheumatoid factor in the blood. A positive test may help with confirming a diagnosis or in predicting how severe disease will become. It is rarely positive in children unless they have RF-positive polyarthritis. A positive result can mean a greater risk of severe disease so aggressive treatment is often used.

Rheumatologist: A physician who specializes in the diagnosis, treatment and prevention or arthritis and other rheumatic disorders.

Sclerodactyly: Localized scleroderma of the fingers or toes.

Scleroderma: A chronic hardening and thickening of the skin. Scleroderma is rare in children. There are two general categories of scleroderma: localized scleroderma, which mainly affects the skin, and systemic scleroderma (sclerosis), which may affect the skin as well as other parts of the body.

Social worker: A licensed professional who assists people in need by helping them capitalized on their own resources and connecting them with social services such as home nursing care or vocational rehabilitation.

Soft tissue release: Surgery in which tight tissues are cut and repaired to allow the joint to return to its normal position.

Spondyloarthropathies: A group of diseases that involve the spine. These include ankylosing spondylitis, seronegative enthesopathy and arthropathy syndrome (SEA syndrome), arthritis associated with inflammatory bowel disease, reactive arthritis and Reiter's syndrome. These diseases occur more often in males than females.

Synovectomy: Surgery in which the diseased lining of the joint, the synovial membrane, or a portion on the lining is removed.

Systemic lupus erythematosus (SLE or lupus): A rheumatic disease involving the skin, joints, muscles and sometimes internal organs. Lupus is a chronic inflammatory disease characterized by fever and rash that come and go. Most children with lupus develop the disease during adolescence.

Temporomandibular joint (TMJ): the joint in front of the ears, where the lower jaw connects to the base of the skull. Arthritis may affect this joint in the same way it does others, by causing pain, stiffness and altered growth.

Therapist: A medical professional that specializes in providing a certain type of therapy. This could include but is not limited to physical therapy, occupational therapy or mental health assistance.

Vasculitis: Diseases characterized by inflammation of the blood vessels. Forms of vasculitis include Henoch-Schonlein purpura (HSP), polyarteritis nodosa, Kawasaki disease, Wegener's granulomatosis, Takayasu's arteritis and Behcet's syndrome. These conditions can be primary childhood diseases or features of other syndromes such as juvenile dermatomyositis and lupus.

Appendix

Arthritis Foundation Resources

The Arthritis Foundation is the only national voluntary health organization that works for the 46 million adults and 300,000 children in the U.S. living with arthritis and related diseases. With 150 offices nationwide, the Arthritis Foundation has many valuable resources to offer families of children with arthritis.

To find an Arthritis Foundation office near you, visit **www.arthritis.org** or call **800-283-7800**.

Programs and Services

Many local offices of the Arthritis Foundation offer a variety of programs for families, from support groups to family outings and special events. Contact your local office or visit **www.arthritis.org/ja-alliance-main** to see a listing of programs available in your area.

SUMMER CAMPS: Many Arthritis Foundation offices run summer camps for kids with juvenile arthritis. These camps are a great way for your child to meet other kids with arthritis while having fun in an environment tailored with their needs in mind. Contact your local office, or visit **www.arthritis. org/ja-alliance_main** to see a listing of camps across the county.

PEN PAL PROGRAM: Kids can connect across the miles through the Arthritis Foundation's Pen Pal program. To participate, contact at the Greater Chicago office at **312-372-2080**. When your child signs up, she will be matched with another child with arthritis so they can begin writing or e-mailing to one another and keep in touch throughout the year.

NATIONAL JA CONFERENCE: Held in a different location each year, the Arthritis Foundation hosts a three-day juvenile arthritis conference for the whole family. While children enjoy fun and educational activities with their group leaders, parents meet with other parents and leading health professionals for educational sessions and workshops. Visit **www.arthritis.org** for more information.

Information and Products

The Arthritis Foundation offers a wealth of information about juvenile arthritis.

WWW.ARTHRITIS.ORG: Information about juvenile arthritis is available 24 hours a day on the Arthritis Foundation's Web site. Find the latest news, research summaries and information about the more than 100 types of arthritis. Learn how you can get involved by becoming a member, volunteering, becoming an advocate or joining the Arthritis Walk. You can also meet other parents of children with arthritis on the Arthritis Foundation message boards.

ARTHRITIS ANSWERS: Call toll-free at **800-283-7800** for 24-hour automated information about arthritis and Arthritis Foundation resources. Trained volunteers and staff are also available at your local Arthritis Foundation office to answer questions and refer you to physicians and other resources. Or e-mail your questions to **help@arthritis.org**.

BROCHURES: The Arthritis Foundation offers more than 60 brochures containing concise, easy-to-read information on a number of topics, including specific disease types, treatments and self-management techniques. Of special interest to parents of children with arthritis are two brochures— *Arthritis in Children* and *When Your Student Has Arthritis*, a brochure intended for school staff. Single copies are available FREE at **www.arthritis.org** or by calling **800-283-7800**.

BOOKS AND VIDEOS: The Arthritis Foundation publishes a variety of books on arthritis and related topics to help readers understand and manage their disease, live a healthier life and cope with the emotional challenges that come with chronic illness. Order books and videos directly at **www.arthritis.org** or by calling **800-283-7800**.

ARTHRITIS TODAY: This award-winning bimonthly magazine provides the latest information on research, new treatments, trends and tips from experts and other readers. A one-year subscription to *Arthritis Today* is included when you become a member of the Arthritis Foundation. Annual membership is $20 and helps fund research and programs for arthritis. Visit **www.arthritis.org** or call **800-283-7800**.

KIDS GET ARTHRITIS TOO: The only national print publication for families of children with arthritis, this newsletter is published six times a year, providing parents with the latest news in diagnosis, treatment and research of juvenile arthritis. Each issue also features inspirational stories of children living with the disease as well as tips for coping and juggling the demands of family life. An archive of past issues is located on the Arthritis Foundation's Web site at **www.arthritis.org/ja-kgat**. This newsletter is funded by an educational grant from Amgen/Wyeth and is FREE. To subscribe, visit **www.arthritis.org** or call **800-283-7800**.

Appendix

Additional Resources

··

MEDICAL ORGANIZATIONS

American Academy of Pediatrics
847-434-4000
www.aap.org

American College of Rheumatology
404-633-3777
www.rheumatology.org

American Uveitis Society
www.uveitissociety.org

Food and Drug Administration
888-463-6332
www.fda.gov

Juvenile Scleroderma Network
310-519-9511
866-338-5892
www.jsdn.org

Lupus Foundation of America
202-349-1155
800-558-0121
www.lupus.org

National Fibromyalgia Association
714-921-0150
www.fmaware.org

National Institute of Arthritis and Musculoskeletal and Skin Diseases (NIAMS) Information Clearinghouse
301-495-4484
877-226-4267
www.niams.nih.gov

National Psoriasis Foundation
503-244-7404
800-723-9166
www.psoriasis.org/home

Spondylitis Association of America
818-981-1616
800-777-8189
www.spondylitis.org

············

MEDICAL STUDIES

Goldmuntz, E and White, P. Juvenile Idiopathic Arthritis: A Review for the Pediatrician. *Pediatrics in Review.* 2006; 27: c24-c32.

Petty, RE et al. International League of Associations for Rheumatology Classification of Juvenile Idiopathic Arthritis, Second Revision, Edmonton. 2001: J Rheumatol. 2004; 31 (2): 390-392.

Ravelli, A and Martini, A. Juvenile idiopathic arthritis. *Lancet.* 2007; 369: 767–778.

Sacks, J. et al. Prevalence of and Annual Ambulatory Health Care Visits for Pediatric Arthritis and Other Rheumatologic Conditions in the United States in 2001–2004. *Arthritis & Rheumatism.* 2007; 57: 1439–1445.

U.S. Dept. of Health & Human Services: "The Pediatric Rheumatology Workforce: A Study of the Supply and Demand for Pediatric Rheumatologists" 2007: ftp://ftp.hrsa.gov/bhpr/workforce/ped_rheum.pdf

············

COMPLEMENTARY MEDICINE

Foltz-Gray, Dorothy. *Alternative Treatments for Arthritis.* Atlanta: Arthritis Foundation, 2007.

National Center for Complementary and Alternative Medicine (NCCAM): 888-644-6226; http://nccam.nih.gov

"Rheumatoid Arthritis and Complementary and Alternative Medicine," published by NCCAM: http://nccam.nih.gov/health/RA

············

MEDICAL TEXTBOOK

Cassidy, J., and R. Petty. *Textbook of Pediatric Rheumatology*, 5th ed. Philadelphia: Saunders, 2005. This textbook, written for physicians, covers the full spectrum of rheumatic disease.

············

CLINICAL TRIALS

These sites list the latest research trials and provide some resources related to arthritis diagnosis and treatment.

Childhood Arthritis and Rheumatology Research Alliance (CARRA)
www.carragroup.org

National Institutes of Health
www.clinicaltrials.gov

Pediatric Rheumatology Collaborative Study Group (PRCSG):
www.cincinnatichildrens.org/research/div/rheumatology/resources/prcsg.htm

Pediatric Rheumatology International Trials Organization (PRINTO)
www.printo.it

....

EDUCATION/DISCRIMINATION

Healthy and Ready to Work National Resource Center
www.hrtw.org

Mayerson, Gary. *How To Compromise With Your School District Without Compromising Your Child: A Field Guide For Getting Effective Services For Children With Special Needs.* New York: DRL Books, 2004.

The PACER Center
888-248-0822
www.pacer.org

Siegel, Lawrence M. *Complete IEP Guide: How to Advocate for Your Special Ed Child.* Berkeley, CA: Nolo, 2007.

U.S. Department of Education
http://idea.ed.gov
A centralized online resource for information related to the Individuals with Disabilities Education Act.

U.S. Department of Education: *Students with Disabilities Preparing for Postsecondary Education: Know Your Rights and Responsibilities*:
www.ed.gov/about/offices/list/ocr/transition.html

Wilmshurst, Linda and Alan Brue. *A Parent's Guide to Special Education: Insider Advice on How to Navigate the System and Help Your Child Succeed.* AMACOM, 2005.

Wrightslaw.com
www.wrightslaw.com
An online resource, Wrightslaw posts a wealth of materials on special education law and advocacy.

....

WEB SITES AND ONLINE COMMUNITIES

http://health.groups.yahoo.com/group/jra-list
This forum is designed for parents and caregivers of children who have juvenile arthritis, as well as adults who were diagnosed as children. It is a place to share stories and other information.

www.creakyjoints.org
A Web site started by a college student with arthritis and designed to be a community for people of all ages who have arthritis.

www.pubmed.gov
A service of the U.S. National Library of Medicine that is useful for searching medical journals for published research articles.

www.kidshealth.com
Created by the Nemours Foundation Center for Children's Health Media, KidsHealth provides families with up-to-date health information, including information on juvenile arthritis. This site has separate sections for kids, teens and parents.

....

FINANCIAL ASSISTANCE

Healthy and Ready to Work National Resource Center
provides a primer on private health insurance,
including Health Insurance Portability and Accountability Act:
www.hrtw.org/healthcare/private.html

Healthy and Ready to Work National Resource Center
primer about State Children's Health Insurance Program (SCHIP):
www.hrtw.org/healthcare/schip.html

Internal Revenue Service
www.irs.gov
For more detail, search under health savings accounts,
flexible spending accounts and more.
Publication 502 covers medical deductions.

Partnership for Prescription Assistance
www.pparx.org
A coalition of pharmaceutical companies,
clinicians and other groups provides details about programs
that provide medication for free or at a discounted rate.
You also can call toll-free 1-888-477-2669.

Social Security Administration, disability benefits:
www.ssa.gov/pubs/10029.pdf

U.S. Department of Treasury, Health Savings Accounts:
www.ustreas.gov/offices/public-affairs/hsa

Index

Clinicians, **197**
  assisting, **90–91**
Clinoril, **59**
Clucking, **81**
Cold therapy, **120**
College
  selecting, **179**
  student rights at, **179**
Communication,
  importance of, **29**
Complementary medicine, **60**
  resources on, **207**
Complete blood count (CBC), **9, 197**
Computed tomography (CT) scan, **11**
Consolidated Omnibus Budget Reconciliation Act (COBRA) (1985), **168**
Conversations, facilitating candid, **150–151**
Core strength, exercises to build, **113**
Corticosteroids, **53, 55, 77, 112**
  defined, **197**
  side effects of, **53**
  synthetic forms of, **53**
COX-2 inhibitors, **59, 62–63**
C-reactive protein, **40**
Cushing's syndrome, **197**
Cyclosporine, **55, 56, 57**
Cystic fibrosis, **24**

D

Daily life, **107–116**
  parent's role in, **116**
  tools for, **108–109, 111–113**
Dancing, **129**
Deltasone, **53, 115**
Dental appliance, **82**
Dental specialist, seeing, **80–81**
Deoxyribonucleic acid (DNA), **197**
Dermatomyositis, **21**

defined, **198, 200**
  juvenile, **20, 146**
Diagnosis, **3–12, 131–139**
  blood work in, **11**
  bottom line in, **12**
  imaging tests in, **11**
  laboratory work in, **11**
  medical history in, **4, 11**
  physical exam in making, **4, 6**
  processing, **133**
  questions to ask, **34**
  sharing, **132**
  talking to your child about, **133–134**
  X-rays in, **11**
Diagnostic tests
  preparing for, **30**
  scheduling, **30**
Diary, keeping pain, **102**
Diclofenac sodium, **59**
Diet, **112–113**
Dietitian, **197**
Dingell, Rep. John, **169**
Disability insurance, **173**
Disalcid, **59**
Discoid rash, **197**
Discrimination, resources on, **208**
Disease(s), **197**
  acute, **196**
  autoimmune, **3–4, 23–24, 197**
  borrowing medications from other, **56**
  chronic, **131, 197**
  Kawasaki, **14, 21**
  Lyme, **199**
  mixed connective tissue, **21, 132, 199**
  rheumatic, **25, 201**
Disease modifying antirheumatic drugs (DMARDs), **55–59**
  defined, **197**
  side effects of, **55**
Distal, defined, **197**
Distraction in handling

injections, **69**
Docosahexaenoic acid (DHA), **61**
Doctor. See also **Pediatric rheumatologists; Rheumatologists**
  finding right, **33–34**
Dressing, tips and tools for, **111**
Dudek, Krystal, personal story of, **42**

E

Eating, tips and tools for, **111**
Education, **153–161**. See also **Special education**
  resources on, **208**
  sample letter to teacher and, **190–191**
  school needs checklist and, **192–193**
Education, U.S. Department, of, Office for Civil Rights, **158, 181**
Eicosapentaenoic acid (EPA), **61**
Elbows
  pain in, **98**
  range-of-motion exercise for, **125**
Electromyogram (EMG), **197**
E-mail, **29, 35**
Enbrel, **51, 54, 72, 119, 123**
Entheses, inflammation of, **19**
Enthesitis-related arthritis, **17, 19**
Epiphysiodesis, **87**
Erythema, **197**
Erythrocyte sedimentation rate (ESR), **9, 40, 198**
Etanercept, **51, 54, 72, 119, 123**
Ethnic differences in rheumatic diseases, **25**
Everett, Nathan, personal story of, **169**
Excedrin, **48, 59, 62**

Hospitalization,
preparing for, **89**
House, tools for working
around, **112**
Huffman, Ann,
personal essay of, **10**
Human genome, **24**
Human leukocyte antigen
(HLA) complex, **26**
Human lymphocyte antigen
(HLA)-B27, **9**
Humira, **51, 76, 79**
Hydroxychloroquine sulfate, **55,
57, 77, 115**

I

Ibuprofen, **59, 104**
Ice pack, **40**
Illness, hiding, **144–145**
Imagery, **103**
Imaging in diagnosis, **11**
Immune response, **198**
Immune system, **23, 48, 198**
Imuran, **55, 56**
Individualized
Education Program (IEP),
153, 155–156, 157
Individuals with Disabilities
Education Act (IDEA) (1991),
155, 158, 179
Indocin, **59**
Indomethacin, **59**
Inflammation, **19, 198**
beating, **58**
of blood vessels, **21**
effects of, **86**
over time, **50**
of entheses, **19**
eye, **16–17, 19, 53, 76–80**
temporomandibular joint
(TMJ), **75, 80–82**
Infliximab, **51, 79, 119**
Injections
giving, **69–71**
learning to give, **70**

Insurance
disability, **173**
health, **49, 163, 165–168**
life, **173**
trip cancellation, **114**
Interleukin-1 (IL-1), **51**
International League of
Associations for
Rheumatology, **15**
Internet
connecting through,
148–149
research on, **29, 35**
Internist, **198**
Iridocyclitis, **77, 198**
Iron deficiency, **9, 112**
Iron deficiency anemia, **115**
Isolation, preventing, **151**
Izzo, Sarah,
personal story of, **123**

J

Jarvis, MD, James N., **25**
Jaw. See also
**Temporomandibular joint
(TMJ)**
alignment of, **80**
degenerative changes in, **80**
pain in, **98–99**
surgery for alignment
problems of, **82**
Joint(s)
correcting deformity, **87**
defined, **6**
examination of, in physical
exam, **6**
healthy, **7**
protecting, **108**
range-of-movement for, **7, 9**
reducing stiffness in, **114**
with rheumatoid arthritis, **7**
Joint fusion (arthrodesis),
87–88
Joint replacement
surgery, **88, 198**
Journal, writing in, **135**

Juvenile, defined, **198**
Juvenile ankylosing spondylitis,
19–20
Juvenile arthritis (JA), **198–199**
blood tests in
diagnosis of, **12**
development of, **23–27**
diagnoses of, **3–12**
living with, **93**
statistics on, **14**
as umbrella term, **1**
Juvenile arthritis camps, **135,
147–148, 203**
Juvenile Arthritis Conference,
148, 204
Juvenile dermatomyositis, **20**
coping with, **146**
Juvenile idiopathic arthritis
(JIA), **14, 15–17, 199**
categories of, **16**
diagnosis of, **15–16, 48**
RF-positive form of, **17**
significance of number, **15**
symptoms of, **16**
Juvenile lupus, **20**
Juvenile psoriatic arthritis, **20**
Juvenile rheumatoid arthritis
(JRA), **199**. See also **Juvenile
idiopathic arthritis (JIA)**
Affected Sib-Pair
Registry, **24**
dropping of term, **14–15**
polyarticular, **25**
Juvenile scleroderma, **20–21**
localized, **20–21**
systemic form, **21**
Juvenile Scleroderma
Network, **206**
Juvenile
spondyloarthropathies, **19**

A Parent's Best Friend.

Up-to-date Information on Juvenile Arthritis

"The **best** and **easiest** way to stay current"

"**Detailed** and deep coverage"

"Helps me make the **right decisions** for my daughter"

"Provides **solutions**"

"**Current** Information that's easy to read"

"Keeps me **in tune** with what I should be doing"

"Makes me feel **connected**"

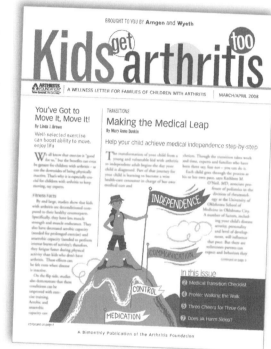

When you subscribe to this FREE newsletter, you'll get the latest news on treatments and research delivered to your home, six times a year. Each issue is chock-full of expert advice and answers to your questions. Plus, you'll find encouragement as you read about other families.

Subscribe TODAY!

800-283-7800 or www.arthritis.org

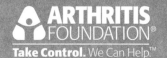